superfood pocketbook
100 top foods for health

superfood pocketbook
100 top foods for health

Michael van Straten

Little Books by Big Names™

To the memory of Kate and her sisters

First published in the United Kingdom in 2003 by Little Books Ltd,
48 Catherine Place, London SW1E 6HL

10 9 8 7 6 5 4 3 2

Text copyright © 2003 by Michael van Straten
Design and layout copyright © 2003 by Little Books Ltd

A CIP catalogue record for this book is available from the British Library.

ISBN: 1 904435 00 9

*Many thanks to: Jamie Ambrose for editorial management,
Ian Hughes of Mousemat Design for jacket and text design,
Margaret Campbell of Scan-Hi Digital and Craig Campbell of
QSP Print for printing consultancy, and Ann Barrett for indexing.*

Printed and bound in Scotland by Scotprint.

contents

INTRODUCTION

If you don't think that eating matters, I feel sorry for you. Some people eat to live, some live to eat, but a combination of both is by far the happiest and healthiest path to follow. When I began studying naturopathy in the late 1950s, I was a food fanatic, but I hadn't been in practice long before I realized that most people do not want to be vegetarians or to live on a diet of nuts, fruits, vegetables, dandelion coffee and boiled water. Unfortunately, there was always the handful of health freaks who would have followed any regime if it was horrid enough. But happily, they were the minority who, for some reason, had developed an enormous guilt complex about anything that linked food with pleasure.

Food *is* pleasure. I'm not just talking about how it looks, smells or tastes, but the far more subtle social pleasures of eating together with friends and family – tragically, a rare occurrence in today's 24/7 society. It is the act of sitting around the table that gives children their earliest introduction to social intercourse, the enjoyment of eating and the development of a complex palate which can savour a multitude of flavours.

It's an inexpensive proposition that reaps huge rewards. For example, my mother, Kate, and her sisters, to whom this book is dedicated, were all wonderful cooks on slender budgets who could stretch any meal for four to feed an infinite number of unexpected guests. My mother's cakes and pastries, Ada's casseroles, Sally's chopped liver, Minnie's salads, Leah's fishcakes and Gertie's roast chicken were all relished by a ravenous hoard of nieces and nephews. What fabulous memories for all of us youngsters who each learned about food, cooking and enjoyment from these six amazing sisters. To this day, their memory is kept alive as, whenever any of the cousins meet up, the conversation inevitably turns to the aunts and their food. To them, eating really mattered – and it should matter to us all.

Now is the time to rebel against the fast-food, junk-food and synthetic-food industry. This is the way to stem the rising tide of childhood obesity, the increasing toll of diabetic children, the premature deaths from heart disease, strokes and many forms of cancer. If this sounds like a tall order, it is. But it's also essential at a time when life expectancy is increasing and the prospect of twenty years of invalidity, illness and debility after retirement is a very real one.

Writing this book has been a bit like *Desert Island Discs*. Choosing the eight records is not so hard; it's leaving out all the others you love that's the most difficult. And so it is here. With room for only 100 foods, what did I leave out? That is a question I spent many hours agonizing over. But here is a distillation of the best 100 foods in the world.

This is not a diet book, or a nutrition book, or a health book; it is an *eating* book. In these pages you'll find many good reasons for using each of the foods listed, but the prime reason for their inclusion is that they taste good. No matter how healthy something may be, if it's horrible, no one's going to eat it. That doesn't mean I have compromised in any way; every single food is included primarily because you'll enjoy eating it. The health benefits are secondary.

After all, the healthiest diet in the world is one that is the most varied, because that's how you can guarantee receiving as wide a spread of essential nutrients as possible. Yet the truth is that average consumers don't eat fats, proteins, carbohydrates, vitamins, minerals and trace elements; they eat *food* – and eating food matters hugely to most people.

I worry desperately about people who exclude whole food groups from their diets on the say-so of some bogus nutritional adviser peering into their eyes or connecting them to some electronic gadget that prints out a computer list of twenty-seven allergy-causing foods. True food allergies are important, but believing you're a sufferer without proper scientific validation puts you at serious risk of malnutrition. And just as the twenty-first-century diet contains too much of many foods and is the cause of much misery, obsessional eating or slavish adherence to some unfounded exclusion diet can be just as damaging.

Eating matters, food matters, and above all, enjoyment matters. So as much as we all have to eat to live, a little bit of living to eat matters, too.

1

superfoods

From almonds to yogurt, each of the following 100 superfoods has a particular health benefit. Everyone knows how healthy broccoli, cabbage and spinach are, but you'll be delighted to learn that every woman should enjoy a glass of beer, that avocados are a superfood for your skin, and that potatoes are low in calories, bursting with nutrients – and they aren't fattening. For a real surprise, discover what makes prunes the most protective of all foods.

Almonds

Almonds are not only delicious, they're symbolic, too. In many cultures, almonds in some form – shelled, roasted, or sugared – are traditional fare at festive occasions such as weddings and confirmations. Of course, the healthiest way to eat them is freshly shelled and natural, but because of their high nutritional value they're ideal finely ground and added to soups, desserts or porridge for anyone who is convalescing or having problems with eating.

The two varieties are sweet and bitter almonds, but the most commonly eaten are the sweet ones. Bitter almonds contain toxic prussic acid and should never be eaten raw, as this poison is only destroyed by heating. Bitter almonds are used mainly to make almond oil. They're rich in protein, heart-protective mono-unsaturated fats and vital minerals like zinc, magnesium, potassium and iron, as well as some B vitamins. Since they're also high in oxalic and phytic acid, which combine with these minerals to carry them out of your body, you should eat them at the same time as vitamin C-rich foods for maximum absorption.

Of all the nuts, almonds contain the most calcium and twenty percent protein; weight for weight, that's a third more protein than eggs. Almond oil is wonderfully soothing to the skin as it's rich in vitamin E and ideal for preventing stretch marks and healing scars.

Almond milk is a classic sickroom drink, used by herbalists for the relief of chest infections and digestive problems. Soak 50g of whole almonds in tepid water then skin them and pound them (you can use a food processor) with some of a litre of water. Add the paste to the rest of the water, stir in a tablespoonful of honey, strain through muslin.

Almond butter makes a highly nutritious alternative to peanut butter and is easy to make at home. An electric coffee grinder is ideal; fill it with a handful of nuts, grind a bit adding a little almond oil, and continue until you have the desired texture. It will keep for up to three days in the fridge.

Angelica

Although angelica is known mostly in its crystallized form as a decoration for cakes, it has a long history of medicinal use. Chinese angelica is a household remedy for women, relieving menstrual discomfort, reducing pain and encouraging the regularity of the cycle. American angelica, sometimes called 'bellyache root', is effective for wind and heartburn, and European angelica is traditionally used for liver disorders and arthritis; it's also a gentle stimulant.

Although used for centuries in China, angelica wasn't a recognized medicine in Europe until the fifteenth century, when tea made from the leaves was used for bronchitis, catarrh, loss of appetite and as a gentle stimulant. Its pungent flavour is used in some liqueurs such as Benedictine, and its iron content makes the bitter leaves a valuable and interesting addition to cooking.

Sprinkle a few angelica leaves into your bath, to stimulate and relieve aching joints. Hang a bag of crushed leaves in your car as a brilliant air freshener; it will also help keep you awake.

Anise

Anise was introduced to Britain in the fourteenth century and taken to the US by the pilgrims, where it became an important crop of medicinal value for the Shakers.

Also known as aniseed, it's from the same family as cumin, dill and fennel, and its flavour and medicinal value come from the essential oils anethole and estragole. The seeds relieve hard, dry coughs and thin congested mucus; they also improve breathing.

To make aniseed tea, crush a teaspoon of seeds and add them to a cup of boiling water. The digestive benefits of anise are legendary, which is why it is often used in the preparation of liqueurs and aperitifs. It can also stimulate lactation in nursing mothers.

Use anise as a delicious flavouring for sweet as well as savoury dishes such as cakes, biscuits, soups, stews and casseroles.

Apples

According to an ancient proverb, 'If you can plant only one tree in your garden, this should be an apple tree.' How true. An apple a day may keep the doctor away, but two is a real tonic for your heart and circulation. Apples are rich in a soluble fibre known as pectin, which helps eliminate cholesterol and protects against environmental pollutants. Two apples a day can lower your cholesterol by ten percent, and the pectin also combines with toxic heavy metals and removes them from the body.

Apples also contain malic and tartaric acids, which improve digestion and the breakdown of fats, so the traditional apple sauce with pork, or sage and apple stuffing in goose, or an apple with cheese not only tastes good but does you good in other ways.

You wouldn't normally think of apples as aromatherapy, but somewhat surprisingly, even their natural perfume can lower your blood pressure and calm the nerves. Medically, they're helpful in the relief of the pain of gout, rheumatism and arthritis, and because of their cleansing properties, they will help you feel better the morning after a night on the town.

Naturopaths have always valued apples as a treatment for diarrhoea and food poisoning. Grated apples, mixed with honey and left in a bowl until they turn brown, make an excellent remedy for diarrhoea. For food poisoning, they're a vital ingredient of the BRAT diet: a traditional method of dealing with food poisoning. It consists of bananas, boiled rice, apples, dry toast, plenty of water and nothing else until the symptoms subside.

The vitamin C found in apples is an immune-booster, and research shows that apple juice can kill a wide range of viruses. As the sugar in this fruit is mostly fructose, it's broken down slowly by the body and helps maintain blood sugar at a steady level, thus avoiding hypoglycaemia and sugar cravings.

Apricots

The health benefits of apricots were first recognized by an ancient tribe called the Hunzas. They lived high in the Himalayas where apricots, both fresh and dried, were a major part of their staple diet. It's known that they had exceptionally long lives; many lived beyond 100.

We now know that apricots are a rich source of betacarotenes, which the body converts into vitamin A – essential for immunity, skin, vision and healthy mucous membranes. Fresh and dried apricots should form a regular part of the diet for anyone with infections, skin problems, with, or at risk of, cancer (e.g. smokers). Because they also contain a wide range of protective plant chemicals, they're important in the prevention of many different types of cancer, especially of the mouth.

Due to their high fibre content, apricots are one of the best foods for the treatment and prevention of constipation. Another major ingredient is potassium, which is heart-protective, helps reduce blood pressure, encourages the elimination of salt, and consequently will reduce fluid retention. They're also a rich source of well-absorbed iron, so they're of triple benefit during pregnancy thanks to the iron, the reduction of fluid retention and the prevention of constipation, all of which can be problems.

Dried apricots make a brilliant snack; they're filling, nourishing and a source of instant as well as slow-release energy. They're a perfect addition to shakes and smoothies, and fresh apricots make delicious, health-giving juice. If you're lucky enough to find really ripe, succulent fruits, remove the stones, put them in a blender and purée. Add some ice-cubes, some sparkling mineral water and you have a refreshing drink. To spoil yourself, add Champagne – much more interesting than Buck's Fizz.

Dried apricots should be bright orange; the darker they are, the less betacarotene they have. Most dried apricots are preserved with sulphur dioxide, which can trigger asthma attacks, so rinse well with warm water before eating.

ARTICHOKES

There are two types of artichoke, totally unrelated, but both with medicinal benefits. Globe artichokes belong to the thistle family and grow throughout the Mediterranean. Jerusalem artichokes come from North America but reached France during the seventeenth century; they are related to sunflowers.

Both artichokes contain little starch, but instead they're rich in a substance known as inulin. The body deals with this in the same way as it copes with fibre, as it isn't broken down during normal digestion but ends up in the large bowel where colonies of probiotic bacteria ferment the inulin. This chemical has all the benefits of fibre but, unfortunately, it can be the cause of excessive wind.

If you're lucky enough to be invited to eat in a French home and the main course is something fairly rich and fatty, you will almost certainly be served globe artichoke as the first course. This wonderful vegetable is a huge source of cynarine, a bitter-tasting substance that increases the flow of bile and improves liver function. The result is better digestion and breakdown of all types of fat, because the extra bile emulsifies the fat into tiny globules – just like washing up liquid on your greasy dishes – which increases the surface area exposed to digestive juices and speeds up the whole process.

Herbalists have long used extracts of globe artichoke (as well as its close relative, the milk thistle) in the treatment of all sorts of liver and gall-bladder disorders. But it's also valuable as a diuretic and can help lower cholesterol levels.

If you're daft enough to end up with a hangover, extracts containing cynarine (or, if you can face it, a whole artichoke) will make you feel better than you deserve.

Jerusalem artichokes are small, potato-like tubers that make wonderful soup and are delicious hot or cold as a vegetable. Both varieties are the easiest thing in the world to grow and produce abundant crops, so if you've got the space, plant some.

Asparagus

This is one of the world's great food treats, with a reputation of being a gourmet delicacy. In restaurants, it's always expensive, and its health benefits are diminished by the addition of rich sauces, piles of Parmesan cheese or far too much melted butter – all of which are sources of artery-clogging saturated fat.

If there's any space in your garden for an asparagus bed, have one. Although the first couple of years take time and effort, the reward of fresh spears, homemade soup, or real asparagus omelettes for the next ten years requires very little work.

Asparagus has been used for medical purposes for the last 500 years, but it has been cultivated as a vegetable for more than two millennia. Although it's helpful in the relief of urinary infections, constipation, arthritis and rheumatism, its most powerful effect is as a diuretic. A natural chemical called asparagine is responsible for this action, as you'll soon realize within half an hour of eating a portion.

Not only will your output of urine increase, but it will have a distinctive smell that is unmistakable (but perfectly normal).

Over a thousand years ago, Dioscorides, the pioneering Greek doctor, used asparagus to treat both liver and kidney disorders, but it took 1,500 years before it was widely used as a medicine again. Although it is a great help in the relief of arthritis and rheumatism, avoid asparagus like the plague if you suffer from gout. It contains a group of chemicals called purines which can trigger episodes and greatly aggravate the pain if you're already having an attack.

Don't waste anything when you prepare and cook asparagus, as the bottom ends which you cut off can go into homemade stock or soups, and the cooking water can be drunk or added to soups and gravies for its diuretic properties. It's also ideal for women who suffer with swollen ankles, fingers and breasts with every period.

Avocados

Almost every single woman I know believes that avocados are fattening. In fact, they're a fabulous food containing a little protein, some starch, heart-protective mono-unsaturated fat, plenty of potassium, and vitamins A, B, C and E.

They've been grown in South America for 8,000 years, where indigenous tribes used the fruit, dried leaves, fresh leaves, rind, bark and the seed medicinally.

Calorie for calorie, avocados offer super nutrition, and the high content of oleic acid they contain makes them a powerful antioxidant. Consequently, they protect us against heart disease, strokes and some forms of cancer.

Puréed avocado is an ideal food for anyone who is unwell or recovering from illness or surgery; it is especially valuable for ill children. It's easy to digest, and a rich source of natural antibiotic and antifungal chemicals. You may think that guacamole is just an excuse for eating lots of tacos, but in fact, it is a dish that provides loads of energy, important amounts of protein, and an extremely valuable source of naturally protective chemicals.

Because they're rich in vitamin E, avocados are important in the diet of anyone planning conception or with fertility problems. Their B vitamin content will help you cope with stress, tension and anxiety. Because they contain vitamin B_6 they're ideal for women suffering from PMS, and should be eaten regularly in the ten days leading up to the next period.

Another totally different benefit is the way in which avocados help improve and maintain healthy skin. The natural oils and vitamins A and E are antioxidant, and thus prevent premature ageing of the skin and the formation of wrinkles. When applied externally, a purée of avocado mixed with live yogurt makes a fabulous face mask for cleansing and nourishing. It will increase the amount of collagen, which helps to reduce existing wrinkles and maintains clear and youthful-looking skin.

Bananas

These are nature's superb fast food, packed with nutrients: potassium, zinc, iron, folic acid and calcium. They're also a good source of pectin, a soluble fibre that improves the elimination of toxins. Sadly, a very common perception is that they're fattening, but this is far from the truth; the average banana supplies fewer than 100 calories.

Because of their combination of instant and slow-release energy as well as cramp-preventing potassium, bananas are the perfect snack for anyone engaged in strenuous exercise. They're also highly protective against high blood pressure, heart disease and fluid retention. Bananas are the perfect replacement for high-sugar and high-fat nibbles when your energy starts to wane during a busy day at work or leisure, and the vitamin B_6 they contain means they're extremely useful for alleviating the symptoms of PMS.

The starch in bananas is not easily digested, which is why they should only be eaten ripe, when most of the starch has turned to sugar.

This happens when the skin becomes speckled brown. Big brother to the banana is the plantain, which should only be eaten cooked, as they're virtually indigestible raw.

As long ago as the 1930s, research showed that bananas were both preventive and curative for stomach ulcers, a fact widely touted in ancient Indian folklore. Traditional practitioners, however, found that the best treatment for ulcers is flour made from dried green plantains and made into a very thin porridge. This fact has now been confirmed by scientific investigation.

Throughout India, Africa and South America, plantains are used much like potatoes. They're a major source of energy and are wonderful to eat boiled, fried or baked, and go particularly well with fish.

Because the fibre found in ripe bananas and cooked plantains is so easily digestible, they help in the treatment of both constipation and diarrhoea. A little-known fact: sticking a piece of banana skin, yellow side out, over a wart or verruca will speed its demise.

BARLEY

Sadly, barley is a much-neglected grain which has amazing nutritional and health properties. The grains contain natural soothing lubricants that have a direct healing action on mucous membranes, which explains its traditional use for the treatment of sore throats, oesophagitis, gastritis and colitis. Barley contains calcium, potassium, and plenty of B-complex vitamins, so it's good if you're feeling stressed, exhausted or recovering from illness.

Lemon barley water is a traditional remedy for cystitis and other urinary problems. Add a tablespoon of washed pot barley to half a litre of water and two quartered unwaxed lemons. Bring to the boil, cover, and simmer for 30 minutes. Strain, refrigerate and drink several glasses a day.

The Latin name for barley is *Hordeum*, and to Romans it was such a strengthening food that gladiators ate it regularly – which is why they were called *Hordearii*, or 'barley-eaters'. The great fourth-century Roman gastronome, Apicius, lists several recipes for barley soups, including *Tisanam* and *Tisanam sic facies,* which were formulated to the Roman medical idea of *tisanam*: barley waters used as medicine, which is where the word 'tisane' originated.

Barley is the oldest cultivated cereal. You can benefit from this strengthening and protective grain by using barley flour in biscuits, bread and cakes, adding barley flakes to breakfast cereals, and using plenty of the whole grains in soups, stews and casseroles. Barley is rich in soluble fibre and other natural chemicals that reduce cholesterol levels and specifically protect against many forms of cancer. Modern research has shown that barley inhibits the manufacture of cholesterol in the liver as well as increasing its elimination from the body.

Pot barley is highly superior to the more widely available pearl barley, as it retains much more of the fibres and gut-soothing chemicals. Although more processed forms do provide good quantities of minerals, they contain considerably smaller amounts of vitamins.

Basil

The traditional ingredient of Mediterranean tomato dishes and an important component of pesto sauce, basil is one of the most versatile and useful culinary herbs. Although everyone thinks of this as a Mediterranean plant, it actually started life in the east, where it is native to India, other parts of south Asia and areas of the Middle East. Basil came to Europe early on, and is mentioned by the classical writers of the first two centuries. In fact, the name 'basil' is derived from the Greek *basilikon phuton*, which means 'a kingly herb'.

A variety called holy basil is considered sacred by the Hindus, and in Christianity it is believed to have appeared growing around Christ's tomb after the Resurrection. You'll often find it growing wild around remote churches in Greece, where it's sometimes used to prepare holy water.

The leaves contain volatile oils, especially linalool, limonene and estragole, which account for the medicinal properties of this herb. It relieves flatulence, is an aid to digestion, and its antiseptic properties are said to benefit acne.

If you want a good night's sleep, there's nothing better than the delicate flavour of basil. It's a mild sedative and acts as the perfect evening snack for insomniacs. Simply tear up three or four leaves into small pieces, and add to a sandwich of lettuce and tomato.

There are a number of different varieties, all with slightly different flavours: peppermint, lemon, cinnamon, purple and bush basil. It's really worth growing your own because the flavour of dried basil doesn't even come close to the real thing freshly picked from your window box, garden or greenhouse.

In the Provence region of France, pesto is known as *pistou*, and there is nothing more calming or relaxing at the end of a really stressful day than a bowl of traditional *soupe ou pistou*. Any decent French cookery book will give you the recipe.

If you're having a barbecue, try rubbing exposed skin with a basil leaf – it's a great insect repellent.

Bay leaves

Laurus nobilis is the Latin name for the bay tree. Dedicated to Apollo and used in crowns awarded to emperors, scholars and athletes, this is a prized herb.

Traditional in French *bouquet garni*, the leaves have antiseptic properties, improve digestion and impart flavour. They're a wonderful addition to most soups, stews and casseroles, and indispensable in marinades. They're also great as flavour enhancers in milk-based puddings – but make sure you remove them before eating.

The leaves contain the volatile oils geraniol, cineole and eugenol, and when used in recipes they stimulate digestive juices and improve nutrient absorption from food. This is a particularly good herb for anyone recovering from serious illness as it helps optimize nutrition.

Do try growing one of these evergreens in a sheltered spot in your garden, as the fresh leaves contain more of the essential oils and have a much more subtle flavour.

BEAN SPROUTS

Bean sprouts supply abundant vitamins and minerals. They're cheap, easy to grow and guaranteed free of chemicals if you do it yourself. I always think of sprouted beans (and seeds, too, for that matter) as 'future foods'. Inside the bean are all the nutrients needed to trigger the growth of the next generation of plants.

Sprouting increases the amount of available vitamins. Vitamin B_2 in oats was increased by 2,000 percent by the time green leaves appeared, B_6 was up 500 percent, and folic acid 600 percent. Sprouted wheat contained 600 percent more vitamin C than wheat grain.

Aduki, mung and soya beans, chickpeas, barley and wheat are all easy to grow at home. Soak in warm water for twelve hours. Drain, put in a jam jar, and cover with muslin. Keep the jar in a warm, dark place. Rinse twice a day and enjoy your delicious, nutrient-packed harvest. If you want to be posh, you can buy special sprouting kits.

BEANS

Dried beans or pulses are part of the legume family of plants and the second-largest group of foods forming man's diet. They're low in fat and salt, cholesterol-free, and a rich source of proteins, starches, vitamins, minerals and fibre. They're also cheap and can be stored for long periods. Pound for pound, they contain almost as much protein as fillet steak – at a fraction of the cost and with many more health benefits.

Beans help reduce cholesterol in the blood and are rich in essential minerals, B vitamins and folic acid. They protect against heart disease, circulatory problems and bowel cancer, and they're a valuable source of slow-release energy, making them an excellent food for diabetics. Beans also contain plant hormones called phytoestrogens, which protect against breast and prostate cancers and dramatically reduce the risk of osteoporosis as long as they are part of your regular staple diet.

Dried beans are the cheapest, but many need soaking before cooking, so canned beans are a great alternative; rinse well to remove the salt.

Soya beans are the best vegetable source of protein and can also be made into tofu, soya milk, soya cheese and soya flour. But they also have the highest content of phytoestrogens, and the strongest antioxidant activity, which protects against heart disease and cancer.

All beans are valuable. Some of their individual properties include:

Aduki	Fibre, magnesium, potassium, zinc
Baked beans	Fibre, iron, selenium, iodine (but beware the salt)
Black-eyed	Fibre, selenium, folate
Butter	Fibre, potassium, iron
Chickpeas	Fibre, calcium, iron, zinc
Haricot	Fibre, iron
Kidney	Fibre, potassium, zinc
Mung	Less starch, more folate
Pinto	Potassium, fibre, folate

Worried about the 'flatulence factor'? Add some summer savory for its anti-wind effect. When cooking dried beans, never add salt; this toughens the skins, making them indigestible.

Beef

In early English history, beef was reserved for the ruling Normans; the poor Anglo-Saxons went without until after the thirteenth century. The traditional roast beef of old England, a genuine Aberdeen Angus sirloin or a homemade steak-and-kidney pie taste wonderful and provide essential nutrients, including protein, iron, B vitamins and minerals.

Sadly, these dishes can also be nutritional disasters. We eat too much meat, and reducing consumption of red meat also reduces the risks of bowel cancer, high blood pressure and heart disease. So if you like beef, eat less but buy the best. That means organic. The fat of cattle that have been free-ranged on organic pastures contains conjugated linoleic acid, or CLA, a substance that is almost completely absent in intensively reared animals. Not only does this natural fat have powerful cancer-fighting properties, it also stimulates the conversion of our stored fat into energy, thus helping to control weight.

Non-organic beef will contain chemical residues from its feed and, although they are now banned in most of Europe, it is still likely to contain illegal hormones and antibiotics. Beef imported from other parts of the world will almost certainly contain chemicals you don't want in your body.

Cooking is the key to healthy beef-eating. Always roast joints on a trivet so that the fat drips through into the pan; it's the worst sort of saturated fat that clogs your arteries. Grill or griddle steaks for the same reason, and when making stews or casseroles, remove most of the surface fat before cooking.

If you like burgers, you should make your own, but even then they must be cooked right through to avoid food poisoning. The good news is you can still enjoy rare steaks and roast beef as long as the outside of the meat has been thoroughly cooked. That's where the bugs are until you mince the beef, when they end up on the inside.

BEER

If you find the idea of 'laddettes' swigging pints of bitter unappealing, think again. There are plenty of reasons for women to indulge in this most traditional of all British drinks.

Beer is one of the best nutritional sources of the mineral silicon, which is essential for building strong bones and for the prevention of osteoporosis. Even more importantly, it's easier for the body to use the silicon in beer than in almost any other foodstuff. As little as half a pint a day could help prevent the dangerous osteoporosis that causes more than 200,000 fractures every year – most of them in women.

There's even more good news, particularly for women, as the latest evidence from Japan reveals that the hops used in traditional brewing are a good source of phytoestrogens: the natural plant hormones that protect against osteoporosis. If you really want to strengthen your bones, next time you go to a pub, have a ploughman's lunch and a glass of beer. The calcium in the cheese and natural ingredients in the beer make this the perfect bone-building meal.

This wonderful drink is also an excellent source of B vitamins, notably B_{12}, B_6 and folic acid, which many women lack in their diets. As a bonus, hops have a natural antibiotic action that kills the *Helicobacter pylori* bug, a common cause of stomach ulcers. For this reason, regular but modest beer-drinkers are much less likely to suffer from this problem.

Beer contains lots of potassium but very little sodium, so it's good for your blood pressure. Its high levels of magnesium and small quantities of calcium help to prevent kidney and gallstones, and a pint provides up to thirty percent of your daily fibre needs, thanks to the barley content. It's this special form of soluble fibre that prevents constipation and keeps your cholesterol low.

Beer is nature's tonic. It looks good, tastes good and really does you good.

Beetroot

Ancient Greeks revered beetroot as a medicine and offered it as a tribute to Apollo in the temple at Delphi. Although there's not yet a great deal of scientific evidence to support the medicinal value of the beetroot, there is more than enough folklore and herbalists' knowledge to recommend it. Eat beetroot at least once a week for specific therapeutic benefits.

In Romany medicine, beetroot juice was used as a blood-builder, and in Russia and Eastern Europe, it is still used to increase resistance and to strengthen convalescents. Fresh, raw beet juice is a powerful blood-cleanser and tonic, and was valued for centuries as a digestive aid and liver stimulant.

In the traditional medicine of central Europe, beetroot has long been used in the treatment of cancer, and now modern research is beginning to explain its healing action. Some specific anti-carcinogens are bound to the red colouring matter, and it also increases the cellular uptake of oxygen by as much as 400 percent.

Beet greens are equally valuable, containing betacarotene and other carotenoids, lots of folate, potassium, some iron and vitamin C, all of which makes the roots and greens excellent for women planning pregnancy, women in general and anyone suffering from chronic fatigue syndromes.

A mixture of beetroot, carrot, apple and celery juice makes an excellent treatment for ME, Tired all the Time syndrome, chronic fatigue, glandular fever and other debilitating illnesses. Try taking a small wineglass of this delicious drink before each meal.

Beetroot is best eaten raw in a salad, boiled as a vegetable, baked in the oven or as traditional beetroot soup (borscht). Don't forget the leaves, which can be cooked like spinach.

And don't panic when you go to the loo. I've frequently been called at three in the morning by a patient whom I've put on the beetroot juice therapy to say they're passing blood in their urine or stool. It's only the beetroot's colouring.

BLACKBERRIES

Although cultivated varieties are now available, nothing compares with the taste of freshly picked wild blackberries. They grow rampantly almost anywhere, and thanks to divine intervention, they're at their best at the same time as Bramley apples. The late summer/early autumn treat of apple and blackberry pie comes at just the right time to boost the immune system for the cold, wet days to come.

The ancient Greeks used blackberries to treat gout, and they're a good source of fibre. They're rich in vitamins E and C, so they're useful in the prevention and treatment of heart and circulatory problems and protective against cancers, degenerative diseases and infections.

Their astringent leaves contain antiseptic tannins, so chopped and used as tea they're an excellent mouthwash for gum problems and infections such as gingivitis, as well as an effective gargle for sore throats. An ounce of dried leaves in a pint of boiling water is an excellent remedy for diarrhoea; two cups a day is usually sufficient. A poultice of leaves macerated in boiling water and left to cool is a traditional remedy for scalds; the tannins act as an antiseptic and prevent secondary infection.

Try treating yourself to blackberry cordial with nutmeg, cloves and a little brandy for a real boost when you're feeling down. They're also an extremely good way of lowering high temperatures; simply soak fresh berries in apple cider vinegar for three days, strain through a sieve, add a pound of sugar for each pint of liquid, boil for five minutes and bottle when cool. One teaspoon of this mixture in a glass of water helps reduce fever and quench the thirst in adults and children.

Gathering blackberries used to be a great family outing that marked the end of summer but, sadly, few people seem to bother these days. The wild blackberry is food for free and collecting them is great exercise – but don't pick them from roadside hedges where they're likely to be contaminated by traffic fumes.

BLACKCURRANTS

The blackcurrant gets its proper name, *Ribes*, from an ancient Arabic word and has been used as both food and medicine for many centuries. These tart, uniquely flavoured berries are an exceptionally rich source of vitamin C, containing four times as much as an equivalent weight of oranges; one ounce will give you 60mg of this vital vitamin. The vitamin C in blackcurrants is particularly stable. French studies have shown that other substances in the fruit inhibit its oxidation and a syrup of blackcurrants loses only fifteen percent of its vitamin C in a year.

It's vitamin C that most people think of as the real medicinal value of this tiny berry, and it is a powerful antioxidant, protecting against heart disease, circulatory problems and all manner of infections. But blackcurrants also contain substantial amounts of potassium and very little sodium, so they help with water retention and are useful in the treatment of high blood pressure.

Pigments called anthocyanosides in their purple-black skins are antibacterial and have an anti-inflammatory action, which is why slowly sipped blackcurrant juice is an effective folk remedy for sore throats. To make it at home, simmer half a cup of blackcurrants in two cups of hot water for ten minutes, then strain and add some honey. Alternatively, add boiling water to a teaspoon of blackcurrant jelly. This powerful antibacterial effect is valuable in the treatment and prevention of food poisoning, as many of the bugs that trigger stomach upsets are destroyed by the anthocyanosides.

Blackcurrant leaves have important medical uses, too, as they contain volatile oils, tannins and more vitamin C. Put two teaspoons of chopped leaves in a glass of boiling water, cover and leave for ten minutes. Strain and use as a gargle for sore throats or as a mouthwash for painful ulcers. Two cups a day help relieve stress and anxiety as they affect the adrenal glands, stimulating the sympathetic nervous system.

BLUEBERRIES

Blueberries grow as a small shrub with greenish berries that turn a rich purple as they ripen. Distinguishing between various members of this family is not always easy, but cranberries are very close relatives. Other members include bilberries, whortleberries, huckleberries and whinberries.

Blueberries are one of the most powerful health-protective foods. They help protect every cell in the body by their ability to neutralize damaging free-radical chemicals that are by-products of our own chemical processes and also the result of pollution. Thankfully, blueberries are now easily available. They should form a regular part of everyone's diet. Please don't just get them in muffins but sprinkle them fresh on your breakfast cereal, add them to fruit salads, turn them into smoothies along with low-fat yogurt, other berries and a banana. It's hard to believe anything tasting this good is also healthy, but it's a fact that blueberries help slow the ageing processes and protect against heart and circulatory disease and many forms of cancer.

Nutritionally speaking, blueberries are not very exciting, though they do contain reasonable amounts of vitamin C and small amounts of vitamin B_1, betacarotene and potassium. They're also a source of antibacterial anthocyanosides which have a tonic effect on blood vessels, making them good for varicose veins. Like cranberries, they also contain vegetable mucilage, which lines the urinary tract and prevents bacteria attaching themselves to the bladder wall. These antibacterial benefits help in the treatment of cystitis and other urinary infections.

In dried berries, the concentration of tannins and the other antibacterials is substantially increased. In Scandinavia, a traditional soup is made from dried blueberries and used as a simple but effective treatment for diarrhoea.

A traditional American folk remedy is made by soaking blueberries in brandy for three weeks, then straining off the berries. A teaspoonful several times a day is recommended for the treatment of food poisoning.

Brazil nuts

Why do we only eat Brazil nuts at Christmas? My guess is that even most of these get thrown away unshelled. What a tragedy! These hugely nutritious nuts grow high in the crowns of some of the tallest Amazonian rain-forest trees. Brazils have always been important in the diets of the indigenous tribes of the rain forest, and to this day they're collected from wild trees that grow in the forest, not specially grown plantations.

Strictly speaking, they are really seeds, not nuts, as they grow in large, round fruits a bit bigger than a cricket ball. Each fruit contains up to twenty-five nuts arranged like the segments of an orange, which is why they have their unique triangular shape. The fruit drops from the trees about fourteen months after flowering, and if nature is left to its own devices, it's gnawed open by the agouti, a large rodent who carries off the nuts and buries them in the ground.

Commercial harvesters collect the nuts early in the mornings between January and March, and hopefully get to them before the agoutis do. Each fruit can weigh up to 2.5kg and drops from around 200 feet with lethal force, but they're less likely to drop until later in the day.

Brazil nuts are high in fat – mostly the healthy poly- and mono-unsaturated varieties – and soon go rancid, so buy small quantities at a time. They're one of the richest of all sources of the essential mineral selenium, which is so deficient in the British diet. This vital mineral protects men against prostate cancer and women against breast cancer. It's also a vital nutrient to ensure a healthy heart. Unfortunately, the average amount in our daily diet is now only thirty micrograms and the minimum we need is seventy. Three or four each day will give you all you need.

Brazils are also a source of vitamins A, B_1, B_2 and niacin, and surprisingly, they also contain iodine, essential for the thyroid, with 100g supplying ten percent of your daily needs.

Bread

Good bread really is 'the Staff of Life', but most people still believe that it's fattening. This is far from the truth, as it's a vital part of a healthy, balanced diet, and can help weight loss. 'How?' I hear you shouting. 'We've always been told to cut down on starch to lose weight.'

It's the *type* of starch that matters. If you stick to complex wholegrain starches like wholemeal bread, brown rice, pasta, oats and barley, they provide slow-release energy which prevents sugar cravings, plus they're extremely filling, which reduces hunger. They'll also give you protein, B vitamins, vitamin E, minerals and fibre.

If every shopper switched to wholemeal bread today, the health of the nation would start improving tomorrow. If you can't get the kids to eat it, make them sandwiches with one slice of decent white bread on top and wholemeal on the bottom; it usually works.

Six million loaves of processed, sliced, wrapped white bread are produced daily in the UK. Adverts tell us this tasteless, plastic-wrapped cotton wool is just as good as wholemeal. But is it? Wholemeal contains five times as much fibre, and valuable amounts of vitamin E, potassium, iron, zinc, copper, magnesium, thiamine, riboflavin, pantathenic acid, folic acid, pyridoxine and biotin. You'll also get ten times as much manganese, twice as much chromium and one-and-a-half times as much selenium.

Watch out for salt in commercial bread, as most manufacturers label it as 'grams of sodium per 100g'. Multiply this figure by 2.5, and you'll find out how much you're really getting – 530mg of sodium per 100g actually means 1.3g of salt from three slices. Your daily total shouldn't exceed 5g.

The best answer is to make your own, one of the most satisfying things you can ever do in a kitchen. But if you don't fancy all that kneading and pummelling (although it's a great way to get rid of anger and frustration), why not buy a bread machine? Either way, you control exactly what goes into your daily bread.

BROCCOLI

Broccoli is a very rich source of carotenoids, especially betacarotene, which the body converts into vitamin A. Betacarotene and many of the other carotenoids are known to restrict the development and growth of cancer cells, and they play a vital role in the prevention of many types of cancer.

Ever since the scare over US President Reagan's bowel cancer, broccoli has become a four-star vegetable. The American National Cancer Institute advised a special diet for the president which included copious amounts of broccoli. Like other members of the cruciferous family of vegetables, it has been shown to have protective powers against cancer. (Other crucifers include cauliflower, kale, radishes, horseradish, cabbage, spring greens, turnips and Brussels sprouts). According to an analysis conducted by the US National Cancer Institute in 1987, six out of seven major population studies showed that the more cruciferous vegetables you eat, the lower your chances of developing cancer of the colon. Other cancers appeared to slow down as well.

A number of chemical compounds in the cruciferous vegetables have been identified as being responsible for this effect. Glucobrassicin and sinigrin are the major glucosinolates that are present in crucifers, and in response to cell damage they are converted to indoles. In Japan, where the incidence of colon cancer is extremely low, the average intake of glucosinolates is 100mg a day. In Britain, where there is a high incidence of colon cancer, the intake is less than a quarter of this amount.

Because of its potential to increase vitamin A in the body, eating broccoli also helps to improve and prevent a range of skin problems, particularly acne. This vegetable is also a valuable source of iron, as well as folic acid and vitamin C, making it easier for the body to absorb the mineral. For this reason, it's good for the treatment of anaemia and fatigue, and prevents birth defects such as spina bifida.

BUCKWHEAT

Most people think buckwheat is a cereal. It's actually related to rhubarb, and is suitable for anyone with gluten or wheat allergies.

It has a high content of rutin, a substance that strengthens the tiniest blood vessels, and helps frostbite, chilblains and thread veins. Anyone bruising easily or with tiny broken blood vessels under the skin should be cooking with buckwheat flour. Herbalists use extracts to treat hardening of the arteries, high blood pressure and varicose veins.

Buckwheat flour makes wonderful and health-giving pancakes, and is used for this purpose in oriental cooking. The pancakes you get with duck in a Chinese restaurant are always made from buckwheat. It's also a staple food in Russia and Poland, where it's used to make traditional tiny pancakes called blinis. Have them with a topping of smoked salmon, cream cheese or caviar (or preferably all three), and a glass of hot lemon tea if you want a truly mouth-watering experience.

Butter

If you can't taste the difference between butter and margarine, there's something wrong with your taste buds. Despite the adverts, you're better off with butter. It's delicious, and in modest amounts, it's certainly healthier than nearly all margarines. It is virtually all fat and sixty percent of that is saturated fat; 100g of butter give you 740 calories, but it's a rich source of vitamins A, D and E.

Some brands are much higher in salt than others and may contain up to 1,300mg per 100g. In the UK, many brands of butter may be coloured, but they may not contain antioxidants unless the finished product is made exclusively for manufacturing or catering use, so choose unsalted, uncoloured brands.

Unlike most dairy products, butter is a poor source of calcium, but it does not contain the heart and artery-damaging trans-fats produced during the margarine-manufacturing process.

Be sparing with the butter, then, and your food will taste better.

Cabbage

Stir-fried, steamed, braised, stuffed or raw, cabbage is delicious. Only the great British tradition of boiling it to death renders it into a grey, sulphurous, inedible pulp. It doesn't matter what variety of cabbage you choose – Savoy, Chinese, red or white – this amazing family of plants has deservedly been known in Europe as the medicine of the poor since the Middle Ages.

Cabbage is rich in antibacterial sulphur compounds, which makes it valuable for chest infections and skin complaints like acne. It also contains healing mucilaginous substances similar to those produced by the mucous membrane of the gut and stomach for their own protection. Traditional European naturopaths used it to treat stomach ulcers. They prescribed one litre of fresh cabbage juice to be taken daily for ten days: a regime that really works.

Dark-green leaves not only contain iron but also lots of vitamin C, which helps the body absorb this essential mineral. Anyone with anaemia and all women having periods should try to eat some form of cabbage at least five times a week. In addition, it's an excellent source of folic acid, which helps prevent birth defects and contains lots of betacarotene, which is important for healthy skin.

Studies of populations show that eating lots of the cabbage-family vegetables means a much lower incidence of cancers, especially of the lung, colon, breast and uterus. It's the protective plant chemicals that produce this amazing effect, and as soon as the leaves are chopped, crushed, juiced or cooked, enzymes are released that convert these chemicals into indoles, which are anti-carcinogenic.

But there's more. As well as eating this wonderful food, you can use it externally. A large warmed, bruised cabbage leaf wrapped around a painful joint will make it feel much more comfortable, and applied to a painful breast (kept in place with a bra) will reduce the inflammation and swelling of mastitis.

Caffeine

The first coffee shop opened in London in 1652; coffee consumption – and with it, caffeine – has been growing ever since. There's also caffeine in tea, chocolate and cola drinks.

On the positive side, caffeine stimulates the brain, concentration and fights fatigue. It helps some asthmatics, increases the potency of painkillers and even helps migraines. The down side is that it pushes up your blood pressure: one espresso can increase it ten percent for up to three hours. Excessive amounts cause caffeinism: tremor, irritability, insomnia and sweating. Boiled coffee increases the risk of cancer and more than three cups a day of any sort has been linked to PMS, cyclic breast lumps, poor fertility and low birth weight.

Pregnant women and vegetarians should reduce their consumption, as caffeine affects absorption of the minerals iron and zinc. It also increases the amount of stomach acid produced, causing heartburn and indigestion.

So enjoy a cup of good coffee, tea or cocoa, but limit the amounts and don't get hooked.

Caraway

This wonderful aromatic herb comes from the same family as parsley and has been used in food and medicine since ancient times. The Roman cookery writer Apicius recommended it with vegetables and fish, while in medieval times it was used in bean and cabbage recipes. By the 1600s, it appeared in bread-making. Popular in European and Jewish cooking, you'll find these seeds today in breads, sauerkraut, cheeses, goulash, roast goose and cooked fruit, and as the basis for the Dutch liqueur, *Kummel*.

The great medicinal value of caraway seeds is in the treatment and prevention of wind and indigestion, and it's common in parts of Europe for people to chew a few seeds before a meal. Adding some seeds to bean and cabbage-based recipes reduces the 'flatulence factor'.

An effective expectorant, they're a common ingredient used in children's cough medicines. Herbalists have used them for centuries as a mild diuretic and to stimulate production of breast milk. Chew the seeds for a great natural breath freshener.

CARROTS

Carrots contain so much betacarotene that a single large one provides enough betacarotene for your body to convert into a whole day's dose of vitamin A. Though baby carrots may taste sweeter, it's the old, dark-orange carrots that contain the most of this essential nutrient.

Betacarotene is better absorbed from cooked carrots, especially if there is some fat or oil in the same meal. We now know that, like other carotenoids, betacarotene has many vital functions of its own, most importantly in the prevention of cancer. People eating lots of carrots specifically have less risk of developing lung and breast cancer, and greater protection against many others, too.

As a powerful antioxidant food, carrots are anti-ageing and help protect the skin against sun damage and wrinkles. They're also essential in fighting arterial disease, as they help improve blood flow in the coronary arteries of the heart. Russian scientists have isolated a natural chemical in carrots called daucarine, which triggers dilation of the blood vessels and explains their circulatory benefits.

Carrots are a common traditional remedy for diarrhoea, especially puréed for children and infants. For adults with this type of problem, slice the carrots thinly, steam till tender and mix with plain boiled rice. If you've had several days of partying, clubbing, or large business lunches, and you've had too much rich food and booze, give your liver a holiday and try a two-day fast on nothing but fresh carrot juice and plenty of water to stimulate the liver.

There have been some recent scares about the high levels of pesticide residue in carrots. It is recommended that they should be peeled and the tops and bottoms discarded. Organophosphate pesticides are extremely toxic, so whenever possible, choose organically grown carrots. This is even more important if you're feeding them to babies and small children, but there are now excellent varieties of commercially available organic baby foods.

Cauliflower

Like cabbage, cauliflower is a member of the *Brassica* family, and although containing the same cancer-fighting compounds, it provides less betacarotene and riboflavin. These vital constituents are easily destroyed by cooking, so cut the cauliflower into small florets, wash well and eat as a crudité with dips made from flavoured live yogurt or fromage frais.

Cauliflower is an excellent source of folic acid, which protects against heart disease and birth defects, making it a particularly healthy vegetable. It does provide some vitamin C, so it's a good immune-booster, but the white part is in fact the immature flowering head. Eating some of the tender green leaves closest to the flower will increase the amounts of vitamin C, betacarotene and folic acid that you get.

Because cauliflower is one of the very few vegetables most children will eat, serving it as cauliflower cheese provides all the benefits of the vegetable plus a huge boost of bone-building calcium many children don't get enough of.

Cayenne pepper

People are always surprised about the medicinal benefits of this fiery chilli. It's a member of the *Capsicum* family, which includes all the other peppers. Cayenne has little nutritional value, but it has been used as medicine for at least 2,000 years in Asia and South America, as well as in Europe since the Middle Ages.

The most important constituent is capsaicin, a powerful circulatory stimulant. This makes cayenne an effective treatment for the relief of cold hands and feet, chilblains, Raynaud's disease and all kinds of joint pain. As well as adding it to your food, it's now available in cream form, so you can use it for external application. Alternatively, when you go for a winter walk in the cold and damp and your feet end up feeling like two blocks of ice, just sprinkle a little cayenne powder into your socks to warm them.

Make sure you wash your hands thoroughly after using cayenne, and never touch eyes or other sensitive bits with cayenne on your fingers.

CELERY

Because 100g of celery contains only seven calories, from a dieter's point of view it's a true 'negative food', because you burn more calories chewing, swallowing, digesting and getting rid of this plant than you get from eating it. As a vegetable, it's also a very poor source of nutrients as it's just over ninety-five percent water, although it does provide a modest amount of potassium. If you eat the unblanched, dark-green variety and the leaves, you'll also get some betacarotene and a little folic acid.

The real value of celery is its delicious flavour and powerful medicinal effects. Hippocrates, the father of modern medicine, used celery to make remedies for nervous patients – and how right he was. Essential oils extracted from the seed have a strong calming influence on the central nervous system and they also help lower blood pressure.

Wild celery was also highly valued by the Romans for its medicinal value, but cultivated varieties were developed by Italian gardeners in the Po Valley during the Middle Ages. It was only introduced to Britain as a vegetable towards the end of the seventeenth century, since when both wild and cultivated varieties have been popular with herbalists.

Celery is a traditional diuretic and helps in the elimination of water. This makes it good to eat if you have puffy hands and feet or swollen breasts just before a period. The seeds are also widely used for rheumatism, arthritis and gout, as they help remove uric acid which aggravates the pain of all these joint disorders. They're also a good antiseptic so, along with their diuretic effect, they help cystitis and other urinary infections. Put half a teaspoon of seeds in a cup of boiling water, cover and leave to steep for ten minutes, strain, add a little honey and drink three cups a day. (Don't use if you're pregnant or have kidney disease, however.)

Combine medicine and taste by sprinkling ground celery seeds into tomato juice, or mixing them with a little salt and use to flavour quails or gulls eggs.

CHEESE

Five thousand years ago, the Sumerians were making twenty different types of cheese, and 7,000 years before them, man was making soft cheese from sheep's and goat's milk. The ancient Greeks and Romans were great cheese-makers and their products were highly valued as an important food. In fact, every Roman legionnaire was entitled to a daily portion of cheese. So why, in the twenty-first century, are we turning our backs on this amazing source of pleasure and essential nutrients?

I grow increasingly concerned that many people, especially young women, interpret a low-fat diet as being a no-fat diet, and for this reason exclude most dairy products from their regular food intake. Sadly, this is not always done for health reasons; it's much more likely to be in the pursuit of thinness.

As a source of calcium, for building strong bones; essential protein; vitamin D, to help absorb the calcium; a selection of B vitamins for the central nervous system; vitamin A as a cancer-fighter; and for healthy skin and a spread of essential minerals, it's hard to better an ounce of good cheese.

Cheese supplies some zinc in an easily absorbed form, and 100g has a quarter of your daily needs. Zinc is vital for normal male sexual function. Cheese is also good for children and adolescents, as they need the calcium for their bones. Worryingly, around half of British youngsters don't get enough.

Some people with migraine react badly to the chemical tyramine in cheese, which can trigger attacks; there are also those with an allergy to cows milk. Goat and sheep cheeses make a wonderful alternative, and for both of these groups, they usually present no problems. Most goat cheese is soft and mild, but if you like hard cheese, then the Spanish sheeps' milk Manchega is exceptional: hard, with a full but mild flavour. French Roquefort, Italian Pecorino and Greek feta are among the more strongly flavoured sheep cheeses.

CHERRIES

Is there anything that tastes better than the first cherries of the season, especially as they're one of the few seasonal fruits only available for a few months of the year? It may be convenient to have other fruits and vegetables in the supermarkets 365 days a year, but the best nutritional content comes from fruits and vegetables eaten in season, grown as close to where you live as possible and harvested in peak condition.

Cherries probably came originally from the orchards of Mesopotamia in pre-biblical times, and were certainly highly valued by the ancient Greek physicians. They are a fairly recent arrival in Europe, introduced as the wild cherry from Asia, and though most wild fruits are quite bitter, the wild cherry is sweet and succulent. Of the cultivated varieties, my favourites come from the orchards of Kent. Most cherries in supermarkets are imported.

Of the sour cherries, morello are wonderful for cooking, bottling, juicing and liqueurs, and the acerola is the richest in nutrients, especially bioflavonoids. Wild cherry bark was used medicinally, but the dried fruit stalks and fruits are an effective diuretic. Cherries contain plenty of potassium and virtually no sodium, so they're excellent for anyone with high blood pressure or heart disease.

They're a reasonable source of vitamin C but they also contain significant amounts of bioflavonoids and other plant chemicals, which make them pretty near the top of the list of protective antioxidant foods. It is the ellagic acid content that adds extra value to their anti-cancer properties.

In folk medicine, cherries have been used for the relief of arthritis and gout, and dried cherry stones make the most wonderful hot bag for muscular pain, joint disorders and stomach ache. Although there is no scientific evidence for this, anecdotal stories are legion, and even if they don't help, they can't hurt and they taste delicious.

CHESTNUTS

Apart from stuffing the turkey at Christmas and maybe roasting a few on the fire, chestnuts are a much under-used and underrated food. As far back as prehistoric times they were eaten by the earliest hunter-gatherers, and to this day they are still regarded as staple foods in some parts of the world, particularly in southern Italy.

Unfortunately, they produce poor crops in Britain and they must not be confused with the poisonous horse chestnut used by herbalists. They must be cooked first, but you can then add them to sweet and savoury dishes, vegetables, soups or stuffings. Try cooking a few with Brussels sprouts or adding them to broccoli-and-Stilton soup.

Unlike most other nuts, chestnuts contain virtually no fat and only 170 calories per 100g. Because they're high in starch, they can be dried and ground into excellent gluten-free flour. There's not much protein, but they do contain B vitamins, thiamine (B_1), riboflavin (B_2), pyridoxine (B_6) and potassium.

CHICKPEAS

Chickpeas, like all the pulses, are an amazing food. They're cheap, filling, versatile, easy to use and delicious. You can buy them canned, whole, split or ground into flour.

If you're using dried beans, they need to be soaked in cold water for six hours, then rinsed well before cooking. Canned chickpeas are already cooked and ready to eat, but they must be strained and rinsed thoroughly to remove the salt. Add canned chickpeas to recipes at the end of cooking; otherwise they turn into mush.

Never add salt when cooking chickpeas, as this toughens the skins and makes them more difficult to digest; it's best to season them after cooking. They're great in soups, stews and casseroles and extremely popular in Middle Eastern cooking, where they are the basic ingredient of hummus and falafel.

This pulse has a unique savoury, nutty flavour and nutritionally provides protein, manganese, iron, folic acid and vitamin E.

Chocolate

Feeling low and a bit depressed? Eat some dark chocolate. It's delicious and is there to be enjoyed, so ignore the 'food police' who say it's unhealthy. Good-quality chocolate is, in fact, a source of valuable nutrients as well as pleasure.

The Aztecs were the first to discover chocolate, and the cocoa tree was originally native to Mexico. In earliest times, it was so highly prized that the Aztecs used the cocoa beans as currency; only members of the royal family were allowed to consume it as a drink.

When making chocolate, most of the fat is left in and the quality is determined by the percentage of cocoa solids in the finished product. Most British chocolate is made with added milk, but on the Continent the taste is for much darker forms with a higher percentage of cocoa solids. The very best chocolate contains a minimum of seventy percent.

When the famous botanist Linnaeus named the cocoa tree, he called it *theobroma*, meaning 'food of the gods'. A major constituent of the bean is theobromine, which triggers the release of natural 'feel-good' chemicals in the brain. It's these endorphins which help depression and kindle the feelings of romance, love and arousal. Caffeine is also present, which helps make chocolate a mild diuretic.

Herbalists have used chocolate for its theobromine and the stimulating effect on the heart muscle and the kidneys. Chocolate was traditionally used, combined with *Digitalis*, for fluid retention linked to heart failure, and because it dilates the blood vessels, it can also be useful in the treatment of high blood pressure.

Although it contains fat, dark chocolate is a very good source of iron and magnesium. Chocolate supplies useful amounts of protein and traces of other minerals and some B vitamins. But it's loaded with calories: over 500 per 100g. You'll need to walk briskly for two hours, pedal your bicycle for an hour and a half, or swim nonstop for an hour to burn off 100g of chocolate.

CRANBERRIES

Cranberries are native to North America, and for centuries the American Indians have used them for food and medicine. They washed injuries in cranberry juice, and their medicine men made cranberry poultices to draw poison from arrow wounds. It was the Indians who helped the pilgrims survive by teaching them to live off the land. Thanks to the high vitamin C content in cranberries, they avoided scurvy, and it wasn't long before American whalers were carrying barrels of cranberries, just as the English sailors used limes.

American folk medicine has long prescribed cranberry juice to relieve cystitis, and modern science has now proved the truth of this ancient knowledge. Originally, doctors thought it was the acidity of the juice that killed off the bugs but this is not the most important mechanism. Cranberries contain substances that stick to the lining of the bladder, kidneys and internal plumbing, and they stop bacteria making their home in these sensitive tissues. One glass of cranberry juice is ten times more effective than antibiotics. Most importantly, chronic sufferers should continue with their daily glass even after symptoms have disappeared, as this is a powerful preventer of recurrent attacks.

There are pure organic juices on the market, but do be careful with the more commercial brands as many of them contain low levels of juice and far too much sugar or artificial sweeteners; it's important to read the labels. If you're drinking pure juice, dilute it fifty/fifty with water and do not brush your teeth within half an hour of drinking. This applies to any acidic fruit juice, as the acid softens tooth enamel which is then easily damaged by brushing.

When the native Americans introduced those early starving settlers to the wild turkey, Indian corn (maize), squash, sweet potatoes and cranberries, they saved their lives. To this day Americans celebrate Thanksgiving with a meal of turkey, cornbread, sweet potatoes, pumpkin pie and of course, cranberry sauce.

Dandelion

Traditional English folklore warns children about what happens if they pick dandelions; the north country name for this extremely valuable medicinal plant is 'wet-the-bed'. In France, where you buy it by the kilo in any street market, it's known as *pis en lit* – for the same very good reasons.

Both leaves and roots of the dandelion have historically been used as a diuretic and in the treatment of gall bladder and liver problems ever since the Middle Ages. The leaves help constipation and are good to eat in pregnancy.

It's the bitter taste of the leaves that gives the clue to their value, as it is the unique natural ingredients that stimulate the liver and the production of bile, which in turn improves fat digestion. The leaves are rich in vitamins A and C, as well as iron.

So leave them in the garden and use young leaves tossed in extra-virgin olive oil with bits of crispy bacon: a traditional French salad for fatigue, skin or joint problems.

Dates

Dates have been a vital food crop for 5,000 years, and although they don't contain much in the way of vitamins, they're a rich source of minerals and instant energy. Their iron content, which is little appreciated outside of the East, varies according to variety, but most contain highly significant amounts in an easily absorbed form. You only need ten Gondela dates from the Sudan or fourteen Khidri from Riyadh to provide your daily requirements.

This high iron content, together with the easily available energy, makes dates an excellent nutrient for those suffering from anaemia and illnesses which produce chronic fatigue. Bearing in mind the desert-roaming Bedouin often travelled for days with little more to eat than a store of dates, figs and flour to make their unleavened bread, why not add a few to the lunchbox, for child or adult, instead of a bag of sweets?

As a bonus, throughout the Middle East, dates are believed to be an aphrodisiac.

DILL

Never plant dill too close to fennel, as they're so closely related that you may end up with a hybrid and lose this herb's distinctive flavours. The frond-like leaves add a wonderful flavour to salads, fish, eggs and most vegetables. The seeds have a less pungent smell but a much stronger taste, and they are the traditional addition to pickled cucumbers. They're also excellent added to salad oils and vinegars – especially the cider and wine varieties – as they seem to enhance their natural taste.

Dill contains the volatile oils carvone, limonene and phellandrine, and it's these that make them extremely effective in the relief of flatulence, stomach pain and indigestion. Use the leaves or seeds to make a tea for rapid relief.

Herbalists have long recommended dill to help stimulate the flow of breast milk in nursing mothers, and most babies taste it in gripe water. No coincidence, then, that its name comes from an ancient Saxon word meaning 'to lull'.

Duck

Duck meat is an excellent source of protein, iron, zinc and nearly all the B vitamins. Be warned, though: delicious as the crispy skin is, you will get 29g of fat if you eat 100g of meat and skin, but only 9.7g if you stick to the meat alone. Like chicken, it's even more important to cook duck on a rack. It also helps to prick the skin all over with a sharp fork or skewer, so the fat layer under the skin can trickle out as it melts in the heat of the oven. Served with the traditional apple sauce, it not only tastes wonderful, but the pectins in the apple helps the body eliminate much of the cholesterol eaten with the duck.

Commercially reared birds, like the famous Aylesbury duck, are widely available, but if you ever get the chance to eat the wild fowl, take it. The flavour is slightly stronger, but the fat content is much, much less.

Eggs

Eggs are the ultimate protein. Ninety percent is utilized by the body, compared with only sixty-seven percent from steak and thirty percent from lentils. They're also a wonderful source of zinc and vitamins A, B, D and E.

One of the most important substances in egg yolk is lecithin, which is vital as part of many of the body's metabolic processes, including the dispersal of dangerous fat deposits and cholesterol. Lecithin prevents the development of heart disease as well as the formation of gallstones, and also encourages speedy conversion of body fats into energy.

Because of their high lecithin content, eggs are an important brain food, contributing not only to memory and concentration, but also to good mental and emotional status.

Modern man's obsession with cholesterol means that people have drastically cut down on the number of eggs they eat and go to ridiculous lengths like making disgusting omelettes from one whole egg and three egg whites. Yet there is a big difference between dietary cholesterol and blood cholesterol. The body manufactures cholesterol when you eat saturated animal fats, but the cholesterol in eggs *does not add* to the circulating blood levels; it is only a factor in people who already have extremely high cholesterol or suffer from hereditary diseases which mean they make too much of their own.

You'll be happy to know that the World Health Organization advises a maximum of ten eggs a week. Factory-farmed battery eggs should be avoided as they are much more likely to be infected with salmonella and contain chemical additives that are added to the feed. Always choose organic hens eggs.

Duck and goose eggs are also delicious, but they need to be thoroughly cooked. Hard-boiled quails eggs with a little celery salt are also a wonderful treat. If you want the ultimate 'eggstacy', try gulls eggs for the most delicious, creamy-textured yolks.

FENNEL

Fennel has been used by the Greeks, Romans, Anglo-Saxons and the American Puritans. It was a diet aid for Roman women, while the Puritans nibbled a handful of seeds to stave off hunger during their extremely long church services.

Tea made from the crushed seeds is a good expectorant for coughs and bronchitis, and this herb also relieves flatulence, improves digestion and stimulates the liver. Fennel is a useful diuretic, and an infusion of the seeds is helpful for kidney stones and cystitis.

Seventeenth-century herbalists recognized fennel's value as both food and medicine, and it has long been used to flavour all kinds of fish dishes. Most fennel is grown for its feathery leaves and seeds, yet the stately bronze fennel is one of the most beautiful plants in the herb garden.

Florence fennel produces a large white bulb that is delicious when eaten raw in salads or cooked, as its aniseed flavour is sweeter than the wild fennel.

Figs

If Adam and Eve used fig leaves, they must have eaten the figs – and I never understood why they bothered with the apple. There are many other biblical references to figs, both as food and medicine. Isaiah, for example, told King Hezekiah to apply a fig poultice when he developed a tumour.

Figs do indeed contain the anti-cancer agent benzaldehyde, as well as healing enzymes, flavonoids and a particular natural chemical, ficin, which starts the breakdown of proteins and improves digestion. Figs are a rich source of iron, potassium, betacarotene, fibre and energy, and throughout Asia are revered as one of the most aphrodisiac of foods.

Buddhists, Hindus and even the Romans regard the fig as a sacred tree, and extracts of the fruit, leaves and bark are important in Indian Ayurvedic medicine. The earliest Olympians consumed masses of fresh figs for strength and stamina. Either fresh or dried, they provide instant energy, potassium to ward off cramp and lots of healthy fibre for modern athletes.

FISH

Tragically, the consumption of fish has been declining for years – which is bad news nutritionally, as fish is one of the healthiest of all foods. It's also perfect for slimmers, which makes it even more extraordinary that in a time when obesity is on the increase and dieting is a national obsession, we still manage to eat less and less of the fruits of the sea.

White fish and most freshwater fish, with the exception of salmon, trout and eels, are a terrific source of protein and minerals and virtually no fat. They provide lots of B vitamins, but their flesh contains virtually no vitamin A, D or E. Fish roe will give you as much iron as the same weight of pork chops or roast lamb.

The oily varieties are another kettle of fish as, thanks to the fats they contain, they provide much more energy and much more of the fat-soluble vitamins. Anchovies, whitebait, herring (see page 94), sardines (see page 159), sprats, mackerel, pilchards and tuna contain vital amounts of omega-3 fatty acids which are essential for normal cell function, powerful anti-inflammatories and vital to the growth and development of the brain and central nervous system during pregnancy and breastfeeding. Yet again, folklore is proved correct – when grannie said eat fish for your brains, she was right on the money.

These oily fish are a vitally important source of vitamin D, without which the body cannot absorb calcium. It's these cheap and quick-to-cook foods that prevent rickets in children and osteoporosis in adults.

Two to three portions of oily fish a week are really essential during pregnancy, and an enormous health bonus at all other times.

Few people get enough iodine in their diets, essential for the thyroid gland to regulate metabolism. Sea fish is the best of all sources.

Read labels on cans and avoid 'vegetable oil' as this mixture certainly contains saturated fat from palm oil. Olive and sunflower are best.

Garlic

Garlic was brought to Britain by Roman centurions who wedged fresh cloves between their toes to prevent foot rot. Some of the discarded garlic took root and this wonderful wild plant soon became established.

Some years ago, a strange coincidence turned me into a garlic freak. Three patients told me their doctors were puzzled by changes in their blood samples. They'd all come to me with different conditions, but the one thing they had in common was heart and circulatory problems, for which they'd been prescribed anticoagulants to 'thin' their blood. In the same week their doctors had reduced the dose of their medication because their blood was getting too thin.

Why did I find this news so exciting? Because the only common treatment that I prescribed for all of them was large doses of garlic.

From as far back as ancient Egypt to Greece, Rome, England in the Middle Ages, and up to the end of the nineteenth century, garlic was the most widely used medicinal plant in the world. Bronchitis, catarrh, sore throats, asthma, indigestion, constipation, diarrhoea and even athlete's foot can all be helped by this powerful little bulb. But by far the most exciting development in the history of this plant is research into its heart and circulatory benefits. In countries where it's eaten in abundance, fewer people die of heart attacks than in the UK and America.

The sulphur compound allicin, released when garlic is crushed, both encourages the elimination of cholesterol from the body, and reduces the quantity of the unhealthy fats which are produced by the liver. In healthy volunteers on fatty diets it has been shown to reduce the level of cholesterol in the blood by up to fifteen percent. Another experiment showed that patients with high cholesterol levels who were given garlic tablets but no dietary advice reduced their cholesterol by twelve percent in four months.

GINGER

Ginger is a warming, antiseptic spice widely used in meat and fish cooking in the East. In the West, it's also a popular sweet spice used dried with fruits like melon, preserved to make rhubarb and ginger jam, and crystallized as confectionery. It has been used since 5,000 BC in India and China as both a culinary and medicinal plant. In Indian Ayurvedic medicine, it is considered one of the most important remedies, and traditional Chinese herbalists use some of the non-edible forms for the relief of arthritis, rheumatism and other inflammatory pains. Even the Roman Apicius included ginger in many of his recipes for sweet and savoury sauces.

This wonderful root contains zingiberene, gingerols and very pungent shogaols. Dried ginger contains a higher proportion of the pungent substances, which is why it's much sharper and, to my taste, less palatable than the fresh root. Ginger is the best of all remedies for the prevention of travel sickness and early morning sickness in pregnancy. It's not only completely safe for children, mothers-to-be and the baby in the womb, but clinical trials have shown that it works even better than the normal prescription drugs.

It's effective against coughs, colds, bronchitis and sore throats, and half an inch of fresh ginger grated into hot water, lemon juice and honey as a bedtime drink is a perfect treatment for a cold.

As a nausea remedy, you can buy ginger tea-bags, but making your own tastes better and is very simple. Peel and grate half an inch of ginger root into a cup. Add boiling water, cover and stand for ten minutes. Strain, add a teaspoon of honey and sip slowly. For colds, flu or simply to ginger up body and mind, just add the juice of half a lemon.

Most exciting of all are the latest American studies which show that ginger extracts are just as good for the treatment of arthritis as the standard anti-inflammatory drugs – without any of their dangerous side effects.

Grapefruit

As the perfect eye-opening, wake-up food, grapefruit must be top of the list. Whether you like the sharp, tart taste of ordinary grapefruit or prefer the sweeter, more succulent flavours of pink grapefruit, the benefits are the same.

Like all citrus fruits, they are an extremely rich source of vitamin C, and half a grapefruit or a glass of juice will give you enough for the whole day. Grapefruit has become such an important food that it supplies the average American with sixty percent of the daily requirement of vitamin C.

They're also a good source of potassium and bioflavonoids, both important for your heart and circulation. The soluble fibre pectin is another valuable ingredient which helps the elimination of cholesterol from the body. Pink grapefruit is a good source of a number of the strongly antioxidant carotenoids which help protect against heart disease and cancer, including betacarotene, which the body converts into vitamin A – essential for skin, the mucous membranes and the natural defence mechanisms.

But not everyone should start their day with this delicious fruit. If you're taking a particular type of the special heart and blood-pressure pills known as 'calcium blockers', then you shouldn't take grapefruit or its juice less than a couple of hours before or five hours after your medication.

Drugs (like cyclosporin) which suppress the immune system, which are used for very severe rheumatoid arthritis, kidney disease, severe psoriasis and after transplant surgery may also react badly with grapefruit. If you're not sure, read the leaflet that comes with your medicines or check with your doctor.

If you only drink the juice or prepare your fruit so that you eat the flesh and leave the dividing skin and pith behind, you're missing out. It's these parts that are richest in pectin and bioflavonoids. Why not peel the grapefruit and eat the segments like an orange, making sure you leave plenty of the pith attached?

GRAPES

Grapes contain an enormous number of aromatic compounds – far more than all other fruits. Most important of these from the health point of view are the astringent tannins, flavones, red anthocyanins, linalool, geraniol and nerol. These powerful antioxidants are what make grapes such good all-round protectors against heart and circulatory diseases as well as cancer.

Since the earliest times, grapes have been used to produce wine and raisins. Vines were first taken to the New World by Columbus in 1492, then again by the Spanish and Portuguese, who took them to South America. Wine was an essential part of the Communion ritual, so vineyards were important.

It's no accident that these succulent fruits are what most people take to friends in hospital. They are uniquely nourishing, and help in the treatment of anaemia, fatigue, arthritis, gout, rheumatism and especially in convalescence and recovery from surgery or serious illness. Always wash grapes thoroughly in warm running water to remove pesticide and herbicide residue.

Guava

If you want a taste of heaven, put a carton of natural bio-yogurt, a fresh peeled guava and 200ml of semi-skimmed milk into a blender and whiz until smooth. Rich in calcium, gut-friendly bacteria, vitamins and fibre, this is a real powerhouse addition to any breakfast.

The guava, a relative of cinnamon, cloves, allspice and nutmeg, is an extremely good source of vitamin C and can contain up to 400mg in 100g of fruit – a week's worth. It's best to eat guavas slightly underripe, as they lose vitamin C if you leave them to ripen too much. They also supply plenty of fibre, some phosphorous and calcium, as well as B vitamins.

Guava juice is one of the most delicious drinks around, but you'll need to make your own as the commercially available ones are nearly always 'nectars': a mixture of twenty-five percent fruit, ten percent sugar, and sixty-five percent water.

HERRING

Herrings are a member of the *Pelagic* species of fish, and like their relatives mackerel, pilchards, sardines and sprats, they're known as fatty or oily fish. Up to twenty percent of their weight are fats of the healthiest kind, making them a wonderful source of polyunsaturated and other long-chain essential fatty acids. These have a strong anti-inflammatory effect, are totally essential for brain and nervous-system development in babies and can dramatically reduce the risks of strokes and heart disease.

Around sixteen percent of their weight is protein, they're rich in the fat-soluble vitamins A, D and E, and they're a good source of water-soluble B vitamins. Add to all this a good spread of minerals and you can understand why herrings are such an important food. It's a real tragedy that these cheap, delicious and easy-to-cook fish seem not to appeal to today's shoppers, especially when you compare their nutritional benefits with ready meals, take-aways and the ever-growing junk food market.

In Victorian times, the average Londoner consumed 7kg of herring a year and an average of four oysters a week, these being foods for the poor, just like the cockles and whelks which they also ate in huge quantities. In the early twentieth century, however, most Britons preferred white fish – and it was then that lack of vitamin D and atmospheric pollution which blotted out the sun's rays caused a major epidemic of the bone disease rickets; vitamin D is essential for the body's ability to absorb calcium and turn it into strong bones. Jewish children in London's East End seldom got this crippling disease, due to their taste for pickled, salted and fresh herrings.

Like all the oily fish, herrings must be eaten very fresh, as they are extremely perishable. Turning herring into kippers by smoking them stops the fat becoming rancid, gives them a much longer shelf life and a wonderful flavour. Choose undyed kippers and you will avoid any toxic chemicals.

Honey

Honey is a good example of getting what you pay for. Mass-produced, blended, imported honey is cheap, has very little flavour and bears little resemblance to the wonderful produce of the individual beekeeper who knows where his bees collect their nectar.

Ancient societies throughout the world used honey as an energy food, for sweetening, and as a preservative, and the combination of milk and honey has religious connotations in many civilizations. It's referred to in the Old Testament, was frequently used as an offering to the gods by Romans, and Greeks, and to this day is a popular bedtime drink for insomniacs.

Honey contains fructose, glucose and sucrose, and lesser amounts of maltose and dextrins: all forms of sugar. Thanks to its fructose content, however, honey is much sweeter and contains fewer calories than cane or beet sugar. If you must sweeten tea and coffee, use honey for fewer calories and more flavour. It also contains an amazing substance called propolis: a natural antibacterial produced by the bees to protect the hive from infections. That's why real honey never grows mould or goes off.

For thousands of years, honey has been used for medicinal purposes: both internally as a hot, soothing drink for coughs, colds and the relief of stomach pain, indigestion and ulcers, and externally to heal wounds, cuts and abrasions. Plastic surgeons apply it to reduce scarring after surgery, and it is traditionally used to treat leg ulcers. Modern research has investigated the properties of Manuka honey, long used by Maori tribesmen in New Zealand for stomach complaints and wound-healing. This is now known to be so powerfully antibacterial that eating it kills the *Helicobacter pylori* bug that causes stomach ulcers. And it's even effective against the dreaded hospital infection MRSA, where most antibiotics fail. Naturally produced, unfiltered honey contains pollen grains, which is why it's an effective treatment for hay fever. Eat honey from local hives; the bees feed on the plants that trigger your allergies. Three dessertspoons a day can have a dramatic effect.

Horseradish

Today horseradish is a popular condiment, but it has been cultivated for centuries as a medicinal herb. Pliny advised it exclusively as a medicine, and biblically it's one of the five bitter herbs that Jews eat during the celebration of Passover. The powerful antibacterial and anti-cancer properties come from its natural content of siligrin, which breaks down to form isothiocyanates. The plant is rich in sulphur, and its traditional English use as a condiment with roast meats and oily fish is an aid to their digestion.

This powerful root is a wonderful remedy for coughs and sinus problems; it very quickly encourages expectoration and makes the eyes and nose run, clearing the sinuses within minutes. A teaspoon of fresh, grated root with a teaspoon of honey in a cup of boiling water is a remedy for sore throats, blocked sinuses and flu, and an old wives' treatment for hay fever is a sandwich of freshly sliced horseradish – only for the brave.

KALE

Kale is a member of the cabbage family and is grown for its shoots and curly, greenish-yellow leaves. It almost certainly started life in Western Europe, but it is now distributed throughout the world. With all the anti-cancer properties of the cabbage family and a huge amount of betacarotene – 100g provides almost a whole day's dose for the average woman – we should all be eating far more of this delicious vegetable.

Because it is much less bitter than dark-green leafy cabbages or spring greens, it's the perfect vegetable to use to encourage children to eat their greens. Kale is also one of the best sources of lutein, one of the carotenoids that specifically helps prevent an eye disease called Age-related Macular Degeneration (AMD), the most common cause of visual loss in the elderly.

One of the great traditional dishes of the hardy Dutch is *Stumpot*: a delicious and heartwarming mixture of mashed potato mixed with lightly steamed and chopped kale with meat or sausage and gravy.

Kiwi fruit

These fabulous, furry fruits used to be called Chinese Gooseberries, but then New Zealand farmers perfected them as a commercial crop – and they're now the world's major producer. They renamed it kiwi fruit, after the country's national emblem, the kiwi.

Kiwi fruit contains almost twice as much vitamin C as oranges and more fibre than apples. Just one provides twice as much vitamin C as you need for a day and, unusually, the vitamin C in kiwi fruit is extremely stable. Inevitably there is a decline immediately after picking, but even after six months, ninety percent of the vitamin C is still there.

Kiwi fruit is a good boost to the immune system, is helpful for nearly all skin problems and it's a good aid to the digestion. It really is a wonderful food for children, and I've found that the best way of encouraging youngsters to eat them is to put one in an egg cup, slice off the top and let them eat it with a spoon, just like a boiled egg.

The high potassium content of kiwi fruit is extremely important, as most Western diets are very high in sodium (seventy-five percent comes from processed foods) and very short of potassium. Potassium deficiency and sodium excesses are a major cause of high blood pressure, strokes and heart disease. Just missing out on potassium can affect the heart muscle, cause muscle cramp during exercise and can also be a factor in insomnia, exhaustion and depression. An average kiwi fruit will give you around 250mg of potassium, but only about 4mg of sodium.

The fibre content of kiwi fruit and the particular type of mucilage it contains make it an excellent but extremely gentle laxative. They also contain a digestive enzyme called actinidin: similar in action to the papain in papaya. It helps in the breakdown of animal protein and is a useful addition to marinades as it tenderizes meat before cooking. Kiwi fruit is perfect for the elderly, who seldom get enough vitamin C and frequently suffer chronic constipation.

Leeks

Leeks are a member of the all-powerful *Allium* family – garlic, onions, chives – and though not as rich in the anti-carcinogenic chemicals, they, too, are important in the detoxification process. They are also antibacterial and, as such, contribute to the protection against stomach cancer, destroying some of the bacteria in the gut that change harmless nitrates into cancer-causing nitrites.

Leeks have been cultivated for at least 4,000 years as both food and medicine. Ancient Egypt was once described as a country in which 'onions are adored and leeks are gods'. The Greeks and Romans held them in the highest esteem, especially for the treatment of throat and voice problems. The infamous Emperor Nero ate leeks every day to improve the quality of his singing voice, and in French folk medicine, leek soup was a traditional prescription for all breathing problems.

Famous throughout the world for their male-voice choirs, the Welsh adopted the leek as their national emblem, and they're worn by Welshmen and -women throughout the world on St David's Day. Was it, I wonder, only done to celebrate the historic triumph of their king, Cadwallader, when the Welsh defeated the Saxons in 690 AD (the Celtic soldiers wore leeks so they could recognize friends from foes)? Or was it perhaps to improve the quality of their battle songs?

Although leeks contain only small amounts of vitamins, minerals and fibre, they are a reasonable source of folic acid and vitamin C, and a good source of potassium. They are diuretic and have the ability to eliminate uric acid, so they are an excellent food for anyone suffering from gout or arthritis.

When preparing leeks, most people discard the dark-green leafy parts that normally grow above ground and eat only the white stem. This is a great mistake, because the green bits are a good source of betacarotene, which the body converts into vitamin A.

Lemon balm

Lemon balm (also known as melissa) was used in Greek medicine as long as 2,000 years ago. Traditionally, it was planted near beehives and in orchards, as bees are always attracted to the fragrant flowers.

Herbalists have used it for depression since the Middle Ages, and it's used for the same reason today by aromatherapists.

Made into a tea, it's a remedy for anxiety, tension, stress and insomnia, and it's great for kids, too. Throughout Spain, lemon balm is every mother's cure-all for her children's headaches, tummy troubles and temperatures.

Modern research shows that lemon balm is antiviral and helps heal cold sores. Simply dab them with a strong infusion of the leaves, or crush a leaf in your fingers and rub it gently on the sore; this also works for insect bites and stings.

It smells wonderful but tastes awful when cooked, so add fresh leaves to salads or fish dishes at the end of cooking.

LENTILS

Like all pulses, lentils contain lots of protein and valuable amounts of B vitamins, together with iron, zinc and calcium, though the minerals are not well-absorbed unless you eat vitamin C-rich foods at the same meal.

Indian vegetarians always eat rice or Indian bread with dhal. This combination of cereals and pulses provides all the essential amino acids needed for the body to get complete protein. Lentils are also a rich source of fibre, so they prevent constipation, help lower cholesterol and protect against bowel cancer. If you're stressed, exhausted or both, the B vitamins, especially niacin, make them a perfect nerve food.

Unlike other pulses, there's no need to soak lentils before cooking. And although there are different varieties, the nutritional value is the same whether they're red, yellow, green or brown.

If you've got gout, however, be careful, as lentils contain purines which will aggravate the condition.

LIVER

The ancient Persian writings in the *Ebers Papyrus*, the oldest surviving prescription book, contain a treatment for night-blindness. Simply roast an ox liver over the fire, grind it to a paste and administer to the patient who has problems seeing in the dark. This prescription would certainly have worked dramatically well, as night blindness is caused by deficiency of vitamin A – though I'm sure the ancient Persians weren't aware of this.

Liver is lovely and an amazing source of essential nutrients – but try telling that to the children. Liver pâté or sausage are both quite high in saturated fat, but I've always found it easier to get children to eat these a couple of times a month, as the benefits far outweigh the fats.

Liver is an abundant source of well-absorbed iron (essential for healthy blood) and zinc, which is vital for active sperm and a healthy prostate gland. Lack of iron is a common cause of anaemia, especially in women, and zinc deficiency results in loss of appetite and chronic fatigue.

Liver is also the richest of all sources of vitamin A and vitamin B_{12}. In the mid-twentieth century, injections of ox liver, which contains the most B_{12}, were the only treatment for pernicious anaemia. All animal livers are an excellent source of vitamin A, which you need for night vision, natural immunity, protection of all the mucous membranes and for healthy skin. On top of all this, it contains important quantities of riboflavin, pyridoxine and folic acid.

Health warning

If you're pregnant or even trying to get pregnant, DO NOT EAT ANY liver, liver pâté or liver sausage. When I was a student, all pregnant women were advised to eat liver once a week, but now we know that, although sufficient vitamin A is essential for the baby's development, excessive amounts ingested during pregnancy can cause serious birth defects. One teaspoonful of lambs liver contains a day's dose of vitamin A, while an average portion of liver gives you over 500 percent.

Maize

Mexico is believed to be the original native home to maize. This crop, also called corn, is now the second-largest cereal crop in the world, and apart from Antarctica, it grows virtually everywhere. It is the staple food in many of the world's most deprived areas. It's a cheap and reliable provider of energy-giving calories as it needs only a short growing season, produces a high yield and can survive in areas of extremely low rainfall.

Unfortunately, maize does not contain the natural chemical tryptophan, without which the body is unable to absorb nicotinic acid, one of the B vitamins. This is the reason that the deficiency disease pellagra occurs in populations who depend mainly on maize as their staple food, who consume little or no milk and very little or no animal protein. Though scientists knew about nicotinic acid in 1840, it was 100 years before the link was made between this B vitamin and pellagra, a disease that killed 2,000 Americans in 1940.

The name pellagra comes from the Italian *pella* for skin and *agra* meaning rough. In this condition, after the early symptoms of weight loss, weakness and mental difficulties, the skin becomes itchy and scaly, especially on the hands, face and neck. Sores in the mouth and tongue, dementia and problems with the brain and nervous system follow. If the condition is treated before irreversible damage is done to the nervous system, the symptoms improve within a day of taking the first dose of nicotinic acid. In spite of understanding the causes, there are still outbreaks of pellagra in parts of Africa and India. In the West, it's mostly alcoholics who suffer with this disease.

Maize is converted into many different products: cornflakes, popcorn, cornflour, polenta, grits, and even corn syrup, used as a sweetener. It's a gluten-free cereal, so it's fine for anyone with Coeliac disease, for whom Mexican tortillas and all other maize products are suitable.

Mango

An average mango provides more than a day's dose of vitamin C, two-thirds of vitamin A, nearly half vitamin E, almost a quarter of fibre, and useful amounts of potassium, iron and nicotinic acid. It also tastes wonderful, so it's not surprising that it's probably the most eaten of all tropical fruits. A native of India, its history goes back more than 4,000 years. Today, varieties are grown in Australia, South Africa, and Brazil, but my favourite is the small, sweet fruit from Pakistan.

It's a bonus that anything tasting this good is so healthy and a source of extremely powerful, protective antioxidants. Mangos are medicinal as well; in traditional Indian medicine, the antiseptic twigs are chewed to protect teeth and gums, the bark for the treatment of diarrhoea and the fruit for high blood pressure.

Mangos belong to the same family as poison ivy, so if you're preparing lots of them, wear gloves to avoid contact with the potentially very irritating skin.

MILLET

Because millet is never highly refined, it retains all of its essential nutrients. It can be used as a thickener in soups, stews and vegetable casseroles, or it can be ground into a coarse flour and used to make a biscuit-like bread. There are many different varieties of millet, but this is a much-ignored cereal in Britain and the US, although it is popular with 'food reformers'. It should be much more widely used.

This easily digested cereal is gluten-free, so it is suitable for anyone suffering from coeliac disease. It's high in protein, low in starch and particularly rich in the mineral silica. This essential nutrient is a prime ingredient of collagen, the body's glue that binds everything together, and is needed for healthy hair, skin, teeth, eyes and nails.

This high-quality, protein-rich grain is a perfect food for children and invalids, or for anyone who is convalescing after an illness or operation.

MINT

No one should ever need to buy this wonderful herb as it grows anywhere. If you put it in the garden, use a bucket with drainage holes sunk into the ground; otherwise it takes over. It'll grow happily in a pot, and both leaves and flowers are wonderful to eat.

There are many different varieties of mint, each with it's own distinctive flavour. If you have space grow several, especially *Mentha spicata* (spearmint), *Mentha spicata morrocan* (the perfect variety for tea), as well as ginger and pineapple-flavoured varieties.

Spearmint is the oldest medicinal variety, as well as being the common garden mint; it's best for sauce with roast lamb. It has an ancient history stretching back to the Roman Empire, where it was used as a tonic and mental stimulant, and legionnaires took it with them, like garlic, throughout the world. The Egyptians left sprigs of it in the pharaohs' tombs. It's mentioned in the Bible, and the Japanese have been extracting its essential oils since the first century.

Mint tea is a simple treatment for stress-induced headaches. Chewing the leaves or drinking the tea stimulates the cortex of the brain to improve concentration and creates feelings of inner peace and harmony.

Yet it's as a digestive aid that mint comes into its own, which is why its culinary use with fatty meat like lamb is so popular. Mint improves fat digestion and is an effective antacid, thanks to the essential oils menthol and menthone, flavonoids and menthyl acetate. Peppermint oil is still the basis for many prescribed and proprietary indigestion remedies because it is extremely soothing to the stomach lining. Because it relaxes the muscles of the digestive tract, it helps relieve irritable bowel syndrome, stomach cramp and general indigestion.

All over the Middle East, meals end with a glass of mint tea for digestion. To make your own, simply tear up half a dozen mint leaves into a glass, add boiling water, cover, stand for five minutes, sip and enjoy.

Mushrooms

Thousands of years ago, the Egyptians believed mushrooms were a gift from the god Osiris. Ancient Romans said they resulted from lightning thrown to earth by Jupiter during storms; this explained their sudden appearance, as if by magic. The Chinese wrote about mushrooms in the Chow Dynasty 3,000 years ago, explaining how they were used as both food and medicine. Other evidence suggests man was using them 4,000 years earlier than that.

We should all eat more mushrooms. They contain more protein than most other vegetables, are very low in calories, and are good sources of phosphorous and potassium. Although most of the textbooks state that mushrooms are not a source of vitamin B_{12}, the most up-to-date research reveals they are a valuable source of this essential nutrient. One decent-sized field mushroom (or three button mushrooms) will give you enough B_{12} for a day – vital for vegetarians and even more so for vegans, as other plant sources of B_{12} are very limited. The same is true for vitamin E, which is listed as zero in most textbooks. Again, modern research reveals that most mushrooms are a rich source of this essential nutrient: 100g provides more than the minimum daily requirement.

Mushrooms and truffles are the edible portions of fungi; mushrooms appear above ground, truffles below. Of course, not all mushrooms are edible. Some are very poisonous and others taste revolting. Dried mushrooms generally have a much fuller flavour; although expensive, many Italian, Japanese, Chinese and French varieties are now widely available. For modern food researchers, Japanese and Chinese mushrooms are medicinally interesting. Shiitake boosts immunity, for example, Reishi is good for liver disease, high blood pressure and asthma, and Maitake for blood pressure, liver disease and boosting immunity. Washing spoils their delicate flesh, so brush away any grit and wipe clean with a damp cloth.

Nutmeg

All those wonderful Victorian nannies were very clever, and I'm sure it was no accident that rice pudding was a favourite nursery dish. Traditional recipes always included a good sprinkle of nutmeg: the ancient herbalist's equivalent of a modern 'happy pill'. Rice pudding at lunch meant an easy afternoon for the nannies.

Nutmeg and mace both come from the same plant, an evergreen tree called *Myristica fragrans*, which is native to the Indonesian Molucca Islands. Nutmeg is the inside of the seed, while mace is the dried outer covering of the shell.

As far back as the sixth century nutmeg was an important part of the spice trade and widely used in India and the Middle East. Extremely popular in Holland, it's added to everything from cabbage and stews to sweet desserts. The Dutch took it to South Africa, and to this day pumpkin cooked with honey and nutmeg is served with savoury dishes.

The smell and taste of nutmeg and mace are similar, though mace has a slightly more bitter flavour. The most important chemical in nutmeg is myristicin, which has a profound effect on the brain and is chemically similar to mescaline, derived from the famous peyote cactus in Mexico. Nutmeg also stimulates the appetite and is a valuable digestive remedy for food poisoning, diarrhoea and nausea. In India it's used as an aphrodisiac, especially for men.

The hallucinogenic properties of nutmeg are extremely powerful; prisoners on the chain gangs in the southern states of America used to smuggle nutmegs back into the prison and used them as narcotics to make them feel happy. In small doses nutmeg and mace are perfectly safe, but there are reports of death resulting from consuming two whole nutmegs.

This is also an important spice in Indian Ayurvedic medicine, where it's added to traditional remedies for insomnia, coughs and nausea and believed to promote healthy skin.

Oats

Get your oats – and make sure you do it every day as they're one of the most important of all cereals. They have a high nutritional value, providing good amounts of protein, heart-protective polyunsaturated fats, B vitamins and vitamin E, combined with calcium, potassium and magnesium. They're one of the best foods to nourish the nervous system, as well as building strong bones and teeth.

From ancient 'kitchen medicine' to the twenty-first century, oats have been valuable as both food and medicine. They're a highly effective treatment for depression, and herbalists use tinctures of the plant to help patients overcome addiction to tranquillizers.

The soluble fibre in oat bran helps the body get rid of bile acids that would otherwise be converted into cholesterol. Reductions of up to twenty percent have been measured in patients given a daily dose. It's this same fibre that makes porridge, or oats in any form, the best treatment for even the most chronic constipation. Unlike wheat bran, which can sometimes be an irritant, oat bran works more like 'smoothage' than roughage. Oats have the added advantage of not interfering with mineral absorption, as they do not contain phytic acid.

Oats also have a vital role to play in the active prevention of adult onset diabetes – a condition we are now seeing in growing numbers of young children. Oats have a low glycaemic index (GI), which means they release sugar very slowly into the bloodstream; this reduces the production of insulin and the consequent risk of developing diabetes.

As if all that weren't enough, few people realize how good oats are for the skin. Four tablespoons tied into a muslin bag, soaked in the bath and used as a sponge are healing and soothing for dry skin, eczema and psoriasis. This amount is enough for four or five baths. You can even buy oat-based creams and ointments for local application.

Olive oil

How the world has changed. When I was a student, the only place to find olive oil in the UK was at the chemist's, who sold it in tiny bottles for dropping into ears. Thank goodness you're now spoiled for choice in every supermarket, deli and corner shop. Olive oil is the basis of the Mediterranean diet, which we know dramatically reduces the risks of heart disease, high blood pressure, strokes and many forms of cancer.

Extra-virgin olive oil is expensive, but it is the best and should be used for salads, dipping your bread in, and grilling delicately flavoured foods such as fish. Virgin olive oil is slightly more processed, and regular olive oil may be both heat and chemically treated. Which country's oil you choose depends entirely on personal taste. It's really worth experimenting to find which you like the best.

Using olive oil avoids the consumption of saturated animal fats but it also has its own specific health benefits. The mono-unsaturated fats in the oil help reduce cholesterol levels, and because of its high vitamin E content as well, the oil acts as a strong antioxidant, protecting every individual cell from damage. But there are other benefits, too. Some of the natural chemicals in olive oil prevent the absorption of cholesterol and increase the level of what are called HDLs: high-density lipoproteins. It's these that remove the artery-clogging and dangerous LDLs – low-density lipoproteins – from the bloodstream.

Olive oil is the best-digested of all the vegetable oils and produces the most effective stimulation of the gall bladder. This is important for overall fat digestion, as the bile stored in the gall bladder breaks down fatty foods into tiny droplets, which are then more easily processed by the digestive juices. This makes olive oil not only valuable for the relief of liver and gall-bladder problems, but also one of the most important things you can eat to protect your liver.

Onions

Onions belong to the same family as garlic, leeks, spring onions, chives and shallots, and not only do they taste good, they do you good as well. We all love our fried egg and bacon breakfast, and in one of my favourite experiments it was given to a group of volunteers. Half of them also got a portion of fried onions. Blood tests then measured the clotting tendency of both groups. Without the onions, there was increased risk of clotting, with them a reduced one. So if you fancy a fry-up, make sure you don't forget the onions.

Wild onions are a traditional medicine of native North Americans for the treatment of colds, stings and bites. Chinese herbalists use them as a poultice for boils, and in European folk medicine they've been used for anaemia, bronchitis and asthma, genito-urinary infections, arthritis and rheumatism, gout, and premature ageing. A night on the tiles in Paris traditionally ends with a steaming bowl of onion soup to prevent the next day's hangover. In East

Anglia, thick onion soup was a favourite for treating chesty children.

Onions contain the enzyme allinase, which is released when you slice the bulb. The action of allinase on sulphur compounds in the flesh results in the chemicals that not only give onions their flavour but also make you cry. They're very low in calories, but spring onions especially are a good source of vitamin C, as well as small amounts of some B vitamins and traces of minerals.

Onions are diuretic, both dissolving and eliminating urea, which makes them useful in the treatment of rheumatism, arthritis and gout. Like all their relatives, they are also strong antibacterials.

Onions can even help your chilblains. Simply rub the affected area with a thick slice of raw onion. If you've got a colicky baby, put a few slices of onion in a jug of hot water, strain after five minutes and, when cool, give the baby a teaspoonful.

Papaya (pawpaw)

This delicious and nutritious tropical fruit was originally a native of southern Mexico and Costa Rica. Taken to Manila by sixteenth-century Spaniards, it's now grown throughout the tropics. Today, most of the world's supplies come from the United States, where papaya are grown in abundance in Hawaii.

Nutritionally, the papaya is very important in developing countries, as it fruits year-round and is rich in vitamin C. Papaya is also an excellent source of betacarotene, which the body converts to vitamin A. One fruit will give you twice your requirement of vitamin C and almost a third of vitamin A, so papayas boost immunity and are good for the skin and mucus membranes.

Their most important constituent is an enzyme known as papain, which improves digestion. This natural chemical is extracted and dried to a powder that is used by industry as a meat tenderizer. Traditional medicine men of the South American Mayans used the sticky latex, the juice and fruit as herbal medicines, and it's still common in South America to wrap meat in papaya leaves before cooking to produce tender and delicious dishes.

The leaves are also used to improve wound healing, leg ulcers and for the treatment of boils in traditional medicine. And even the seeds are useful. Next time you eat one, save the seeds and add them to olive oil, vinegar and pickles for a unique and very different spicy flavour.

Pawpaws are wonderful for children and make great-tasting smoothies. Halve and deseed the fruit, scoop the flesh into a blender, add a small carton of yogurt and a cup of milk and whiz until smooth and creamy. For adults, whiz with a little water and mix half-and-half with Champagne.

Canned papaya is widely available, but it is nutritionally poor compared to the fresh fruit. Most of the vitamin C and more than half the betacarotene are lost during the processing.

Paprika

Paprika is one of the most important traded spices. It's a product of the *Capsicum annuum*, which began life, like all the peppers, in South America. The most famous use of paprika is in Hungarian cooking, where it's the prime ingredient of goulash, traditionally the beef soup of Hungarian cowboys – not the thick stew more popular today.

Quite how this particular capsicum arrived in the Balkans is actually a bit of a mystery, but they probably came with the travelling Turks during the seventeenth century. The plant was soon established in Hungary, where the warm summers encouraged the development of the wonderful aroma produced by the essential oils in the plant.

The Hungarians and all the Balkan countries use large amounts of paprika for both colour and flavour. It's rich in carotenoids and contains capsaicin, a circulatory stimulant – though not as much as the hot South American chillis. These capsicums are often seen growing in Spain but seldom in the rest of the Mediterranean.

Parsley

The Greeks and Romans loved parsley. They used it as a diuretic and a digestive, and it's valued for the same properties today. Rich in essential oils, coumarins and flavonoids, it also supplies vitamin A and C, some iron, calcium and potassium.

Juiced with apple, carrot and celery, it's an ideal breakfast drink for women suffering monthly fluid retention. It's also delicious and nutritious added generously to all salads.

It's easy to make your own parsley tea. Put a large handful of chopped leaves into a jug, add 850ml of boiling water, cover, leave for ten minutes and strain. When cool, keep it in the refrigerator and drink a glass every three hours as a gentle, natural diuretic.

If there's parsley on your plate, don't push it to one side but eat it, especially if you've got arthritis, rheumatism or gout, as it aids the elimination of uric acid. Chewing a sprig also freshens the breath after onions, garlic, or too much alcohol.

Parsnips

Parsnips are a prime example of foods that should be eaten in season. The modern supermarket trend to have all foods available from the four corners of the earth throughout the year means that over-cultivated, forced and artificially fed produce ends up on the plate with very little flavour and, almost certainly, diminished nutritional value.

This much-ignored and often denigrated vegetable deserves to be treated much better than it is. It has a unique and delicious flavour and can be used in far more interesting ways than just throwing a few cubes of soggy vegetable into a pot of stew, soup or casserole.

The Romans knew a thing or two about food, taste and health, and had magnificent kitchen gardens attached to their villas. The emperor Tiberius ordered regular supplies of fresh parsnips to be sent from the banks of the River Rhine to Rome.

The wild parsnip has been used for centuries in Europe, where it grows around the borders of cultivated fields and in chalky soil in roadside verges. Like carrots, they've long been a popular cultivated vegetable with a history of countryside use. In Germany, they're often eaten together with salted fish during Lent; in Holland, they're used for soup; in Ireland, they were boiled with water and hops to make beer; and English countrywomen turned them into jam and parsnip wine.

The herbalists Culpepper, Gerard and Tournefort, and even evangelist John Wesley, were all fans of the humble parsnip and advised it for both humans and livestock. How right they were, as parsnips provide calories, fibre, potassium, folic acid, vitamin E and traces of minerals and other B vitamins.

They taste best after the first hard frosts of winter. Mash them together with swede, carrot or potato, or brush with a little olive oil and roast. They're even fabulous cooked on the barbecue.

Pasta

Pasta provides complex carbohydrates for slow-release energy, and while wholemeal varieties contain more fibre, minerals and B vitamins, both white and wholemeal are healthy. The idea that pasta is fattening is one of the longest-surviving food myths; it's what you put on it that makes the difference. A creamy carbonara sauce with bits of fatty bacon; bolognaise made from high-fat mince; lasagne that is more cheese than pasta... all of these are certainly high in calories. But the classic *aglio e olio* – spaghetti with garlic and olive oil – or a simple mixture of extra-virgin olive oil, garlic, parsley, rosemary, thyme and basil (*spaghetti alle erbe*), or a dish of pasta with tuna fish and spring onions are all wonderful meals: filling, satisfying, delicious and a weight-watcher's delight.

Like sun-dried fruits and vegetables, cured, smoked or air-dried fish and meat, pasta is one of the oldest convenience foods. Once made and dried, it can be kept for months and cooked in minutes.

Traditional Italian pasta divides into simple basic categories.

Pasta lunga (long pasta)	spaghetti, spaghettini, angel hair, linguini, fusilli etc.
Fettucce (ribbons)	tagliatelli, fettuccini, tagliolini, etc.
Tubi (tubes)	such as penne, macaroni, rigatoni
Odd shapes	like farfalle, conchiglie, orecchiette, lumache, fusilli
Stuffed pastas	ravioli, cappelletti, tortelloni, canneloni, lasagne, etc.

Marco Polo brought pasta home to Italy from China in 1295. It's made with flour milled from durum wheat, which has a high gluten content, making the dough so elastic. In spite of the popularity of fresh pasta, often made using egg and a softer flour, serious Italian cooks tend to prefer dried pasta for the majority of recipes. Today, there are quite palatable wholemeal varieties available, even in supermarkets.

Peaches

Many food books describe peaches and nectarines as different varieties of the same fruit, nectarines sometimes being dubbed as 'smooth-skinned' peaches. In fact, nectarines are no more than a genetic variation of the peach, and both are part of the *Prunus* family of prunes, plums and apricots. The botanical name for the species is *persica*, because early botanists thought they started life in Persia. It's more likely that peaches first grew in China and were introduced to Persia by early traders.

Peaches and nectarines are now grown commercially all over the world, wherever the climate is suitable. Italy and Spain are the biggest European growers, and vast crops come from America. Commercial peaches are heavily sprayed, so buy organic when you can; otherwise, wash them (and all other fruit) thoroughly before eating.

Nutritionally, neither peaches nor nectarines are really great sources of any single nutrient, and there is little difference between them.

Both contain good amounts of vitamin C, nectarines slightly more: one will give you a whole day's requirement. A little fibre, some betacarotene and small amounts of minerals are also available, but because they are virtually salt- and fat-free, they're ideal food for anyone with raised cholesterol and high blood pressure. Best of all, they're low in calories and smell and taste fabulous.

Dried peaches contain far more calories, but 100g will provide almost a day's requirement of iron and a third of your daily need for potassium. Canned peaches may taste good, but they are nutritionally poor, as most of the vitamin C has gone and they're often canned in syrup that is so very high in calories.

In addition to the benefits of this wonderful fruit, peach leaves are a great home treatment for boils. Soak in boiling water till pliable, press out any surplus water and, when cool enough not to scald, apply as a poultice to the boil and cover with a clean cloth.

Peanuts

I can hear you all throwing up your hands in horror and saying, 'This man's mad! What on earth are peanuts doing in a book on healthy eating?' Well, I'm telling you the truth about this wonderful and highly nutritious food. When I ask my patients if they like peanut butter, most of them hang their heads in shame and whisper, 'Yes...' as if it were their guiltiest secret, because almost every woman I know believes that peanuts – and even worse, peanut butter – are guaranteed to pile on the pounds. The facts, however, reveal the exact opposite.

Over the last two or three years, scientists have proved that the common low-fat diet is not nearly as effective for weight loss, nor does it protect against heart disease as well as the Mediterranean concept of a moderate-fat diet which consists mostly of vegetable fats and oils. Most recently, a large-scale experiment demonstrated that eating a teaspoon of peanut butter five days a week helped the participants to lose, on average, a pound a week.

What's more, the mono-unsaturated fats in peanuts reduce cholesterol levels and protect against clogged arteries and heart disease. Additional benefits come from the high content of fibre, folic acid, vitamin E, potassium and the amino acid arginine, which is crucial to heart health.

Peanuts are also one of the great preventers of adult-onset diabetes as they have a super-low glycemic index, which means they hardly raise blood-sugar levels so that the body doesn't need to pump out lots of insulin. All this protection, prolonged energy release, and a wonderful source of nutrients mean that peanuts and peanut butter should be part of your regular eating pattern – as long as you're not allergic to them, and as long as you choose the plain or dry-roasted varieties over their more greasy and salty counterparts.

Pears

Most people think of pears as something you occasionally stick in the fruit bowl. But this is a serious mistake because, although they contain very small amounts of essential nutrients, they have other health-giving properties which are extremely valuable.

Pear trees are native to Europe, and many of the popular modern varieties were propagated by Belgian and French gardeners during the 1700s. My favourite, 'Conference', first grew in Berkshire, but Williams, Red Williams, Comice and Packham are all popular varieties of this delicious fruit.

Pears are a good source of the soluble fibre pectin, which not only helps regular bowel function, but also increases the amount of cholesterol eliminated by the body. They're a reasonable source of vitamin C, some vitamin A and E, and useful amounts of potassium. For digestive problems or convalescence, pears are an easily digestible source of good calories. There's no fat, virtually no sodium and the fruit sugar is easily converted into energy.

Pears are one of the foods least likely to cause any type of allergic reaction, so they're ideal puréed for babies, and used in exclusion diets where food allergies or intolerances are suspected. However, fresh pears do contain a sugar-based alcohol called sorbitol. While this sugar-free sweetener is tooth-friendly, in large amounts it may cause diarrhoea in a small number of susceptible people.

Like all dried fruits, the nutritional value of dried pears is much higher than that of the fresh fruit. They have a very high natural sugar content, which makes them a perfect high-energy snack to sustain you during the day, and to provide the necessary energy before and after physical activities. They also have high levels of potassium, which also helps prevent cramp during exercise, and they contain significant amounts of iron. Drying increases the vitamin A content, and though some vitamin C is lost, some remains in the fruit, together with high levels of natural soluble fibre.

PEAS

The average Brit eats more peas than any other vegetable apart from potatoes, making them the most popular of vegetables. Sadly, a large proportion of these are canned, and though whole canned peas retain some nutrients, canned processed peas – usually mushy peas – lose almost all their vitamin B and C. To make matters worse, both processed varieties have high levels of salt.

Fresh green peas provide an excellent source of thiamine (vitamin B_1); 150g supply more than a day's need. They're also a good source of folic acid, and supply useful amounts of vitamin A and C. Peas are a good source of protein, but they need to be combined with cereals such as rice, pasta or bread to make complete protein.

All forms of peas and chickpeas are excellent sources of fibre. Because the sugars in peas start to convert into starches as soon as the pods are picked from the vine, many people prefer the sweeter taste of frozen peas, though nothing matches the wonderful flavour of home-grown peas straight from the garden.

Modern technology allows peas to be frozen almost instantly after harvesting, conserving both their sweetness and most of their vitamin C content, and they can be kept frozen for up to a year without nutritional losses. Dried peas and chickpeas are also nutritionally valuable but don't contain any vitamin C. Sugar-snap or mange tout have the same sort of nutritional value as green peas, but because you eat the whole pod, you get considerably more vitamin A and C.

Vitamin B and vitamin C are destroyed by heat, so when cooking fresh peas, only boil them long enough to just soften the texture and make sure you use the cooking water in gravies, stocks or soups. Frozen peas have already lost some of their nutrients, so cook them in the minimum amount of water for as short a time as possible – otherwise, the losses become quite significant.

Peppers

Sweet peppers are a terrific source of vitamin C, providing between 60mg and 170mg per 100g of flesh, depending on colour. The colour changes as the fruits ripen, starting at green, the lowest vitamin C level, and ending as red when fully ripe, with almost three times as much of this essential nutrient. Red and yellow varieties also provide considerable amounts of betacarotene. Weight for weight, even a green pepper will give you twice as much vitamin C as an orange, and more than your minimum daily requirement.

Peppers are very low in calories (around fifteen per 100g) contain no fat and virtually no sodium. They do supply folic acid, potassium and fibre, making a valuable contribution to the diet. As well as the betacarotene, they're an excellent source of bioflavonoids; both these substances are powerful protective antioxidants which increase the body's defences against degenerative diseases such as arthritis, cancers, and heart and circulatory diseases. They also play a major role in the prevention of age-related macular degeneration (AMD), the most common cause of visual impairment in the elderly. This is because peppers contain the special carotenoids lutein and zeaxanthine, nutrients which don't occur that widely in nature but specifically protect the tissues of the eye.

An added benefit of peppers is that the waxy substances in their skin prevent oxygen passing through into the flesh, thus protecting the fruits against damaging oxidation which also destroys vitamin C. Unlike almost every other variety of fresh produce, their vitamin C content remains very high even weeks after harvesting – even more so if they're kept refrigerated.

Peppers, like pimentos and chillis, belong to the *Capsicum* family, which originated in the Americas. Columbus brought them back to Europe, and from there they spread to Africa and Asia. Native Americans have used this whole family of plants for more than 5,000 years both as food and, in the case of chillis, as medicines, too.

PINEAPPLE

'Apart from vitamin C and few calories, there's very little to recommend pineapple.' How wrong can you be! This sweet, delicious tropical fruit has been a healing food since earliest times. Sore throats, digestive problems, blood clots and bruising all respond to some of its natural ingredients, with the added benefit of pineapples being both antibacterial and anti-inflammatory.

In the early 1900s, boxing trainers gave their fighters fresh pineapple before each contest. They were very clever, as they knew it reduced the amount of bruising, keeping their boxers looking their best.

The benefits are due to a natural enzyme called bromelain, which can break down many times its own weight of protein in just a few minutes. Happily, it only attacks dead and damaged tissue so doesn't interfere with the lining of the stomach and digestive tract. There are several hundred published research papers about the benefits of pineapple, showing that it is helpful in dispersing blood clots, attacks the bacteria that cause urinary infections and sinus problems, and may actually increase the effects of antibiotics.

Bromelain has also been shown to be an effective anti-inflammatory, making it an exceptionally good fruit for anyone with arthritis, both osteo and rheumatoid. If you're an active sportsperson, pineapple should always be a regular on your shopping list, as it helps stimulate the body's repair mechanisms, thus helping to heal strains and sprains.

You will only get the benefits from ripe pineapples, and uniquely, they stop ripening at the moment of harvest; after that, they just rot. Pulling the leaves out of the top is an old wives' myth – the only way to judge ripeness is by weight, and if the fruit feels heavy for its size, it's full of sweet juice and ready to eat. Soft pineapples will be brown and fermented, and unripe ones will never be improved by sitting in your fruit bowl.

Only the fresh fruit and the juice contain beneficial bromelain.

Potatoes

Let's get this straight once and for all: potatoes are *not* fattening; it's what you do to them that makes the difference. One hundred grams of boiled potatoes contain only eighty calories. Roast them and it's 157 calories; turn them into chips and its nearly 300, and crisps give you 533 calories from just three bags.

Potatoes were the staple food of the Irish for generations, and they supply fibre, B complex vitamins, minerals and vitamin C. Eating the skin is a bonus, as it contains potassium and other nutrients, too. First cultivated by the Incas of South America, who gave the world corn as well as the potato, it's certain that the Spanish took potatoes into southern Europe, but it was Sir Frances Drake who introduced them to both Ireland and Britain.

The starch in cooked potato is easily digestible, so it's good for invalids, anyone with digestive problems and particularly as a weaning food for infants. The biological value of potato protein is just as good as the soya bean; one large jacket potato provides a quarter of your daily need and also over half your vitamin C requirements for a day. In fact, potatoes account for around half of all the vitamin C in the average UK diet – which is a sad reflection on how little fruit and vegetables we consume.

Naturopaths have traditionally used raw potato juice as a highly successful treatment for stomach ulcers and osteoarthritis. It's simple to do: drink half a small wineglass of the juice four times a day for a month. The taste is vile, but you can camouflage it by adding apple and carrot juice, or some honey. Alternatively, add the fresh juice to any soup just before you eat it, but not during cooking.

If you've got high blood pressure, drink a mug of potato-peel tea every day, as it contains lots of potassium. If they're not organic, scrub thoroughly and add a dessertspoon of coarsely chopped peel to a mug of boiling water. Never use green skin or flesh – they're poisonous.

Poultry

Poultry embraces domesticated fowl such as chicken and farm-raised turkeys, geese and ducks (see separate entry, page 79). Until the days of factory farming chicken and turkey were seen as luxuries and kept mostly for special occasions, Christmas and Thanksgiving. Though wild duck and goose were favourites with the hunters, domesticated versions were still expensive.

Chicken and turkey are now so cheap that they're everyday foods for most people, but the price we pay is the lack of flavour and texture, a higher saturated-fat content and the risk of unwanted chemical residues such as antibiotics and growth-promoting hormones. For your health, and especially that of your children, buy organic. It is more expensive but eat it less often and you won't feel the pinch.

The domestic chicken descends from the Indian jungle fowl and was certainly eaten by the ancient Egyptians by the fourteenth century BC. Chicken contains less fat than red meats; most of it is in the skin and easily removed. In addition to protein, chicken provides easily absorbed iron and zinc – twice as much in the dark meat as the breast, but the breast has double the B_6, which fights against PMS. Before roasting, remove all fat from the body cavity and cook on a rack to allow the fat to drip through.

Goose contains huge amounts of iron, zinc and vitamin B_{12}, but nearly as much fat as protein. To cook, place it on a rack over a large pan of water. Cover with foil, making sure it's tucked inside the pan. Bring to the boil and steam the bird for half an hour, which removes a lot of fat. Then roast on the rack, deducting half an hour from cooking time. Delicious though it is, don't eat the skin.

Turkey, on the other hand, is extremely low in fat, and rich in protein, iron and zinc. Traditional free-range birds have much better flavour and texture, and you can enjoy the low-fat crispy skin.

Never throw away any poultry leftovers as they all make fantastic and nourishing soups which are rich in vitamins, minerals and healing enzymes.

Prawns

Prawns belong to the family of crustaceans that includes shrimp, crab, lobster, crayfish and scampi, and real prawns are native to our chilly island waters. Most of the frozen prawns on the market are imported, and their size varies from the small English prawn to the larger Dublin Bay prawn and Italian scampi, through to the big Pacific prawns and the enormous varieties that come from icy Scandinavian waters.

Whichever you choose, they're an excellent source of protein, vitamins and minerals, and they're extremely healthy. Unfortunately, these crustaceans have had a bad press in recent years, because they contain cholesterol. Many doctors and nutritionists advise against them or suggest they should be eaten infrequently and in small quantities. For those of you who love these seafoods, I'm delighted to say that you can relax and enjoy them with pleasure and gusto. They do contain cholesterol, but it is very poorly absorbed during digestion, and they do not contain any of the saturated fats which the body then converts into the cholesterol that's ready to clog up your arteries. There are many published nutritional studies which show that eating prawns actually *reduces* the amount of cholesterol in the bloodstream.

How you cook them makes a huge difference, of course. Boiled prawns contain 107 calories per 100g, whereas fried scampi has 316. Boiled, they contain only 1.8g of fat, which rockets to 17.6g when they're fried.

Like all seafood, prawns have a high sodium content, so never add salt when cooking or eating them. Prawns are a really good source of vitamin B_{12}, which makes them an important food for those who do not eat meat but are happy to consume fish. They also supply iodine, a mineral often lacking in the UK diet and which is essential for the proper function of your thyroid gland, and calcium for strong bones. They're an excellent supplier of selenium – essential for a healthy heart and protection against prostate and breast cancers.

PRUNES

How dreadfully maligned these wonderful dried fruits are. In countries like France, where food is so much appreciated, they're considered a delicacy, whereas we tend to consider them for one purpose only – and that's the least of their value.

Prunes are the dried fruit of a variety of plum which grows around the French town of Agen, below Bordeaux. The Crusaders brought them to Britain from the Middle East, but it was the Arabs who planted them in France much earlier. *Pruneaux d'Agen* is the name unique to this area, and they are as strictly controlled as any fine-wine *appellation contrôlée*.

In the twenty-first century, seventy percent of the total world supply of prunes comes from sunny California, which produces twice the crop of the rest of the world put together. It is fascinating that this now-huge Californian industry began when California nurseryman Louis Pellier persuaded his brother to bring cuttings of the prune plums from Agen back to California after his marriage in France in 1856.

Prunes are rich in potassium, making them valuable for those with high blood pressure. They're also rich in fibre and iron and contain useful amounts of niacin, vitamin B_6 and vitamin A. They're an excellent source of energy, as they are so easily digested and produce 160 calories per 100g. Prunes also contain a chemical called hydroxyphenylisatin, which stimulates the smooth muscle of the large bowel; it is precisely this characteristic that makes them an effective, gentle, non-purging laxative.

Most importantly of all, weight for weight, prunes are the most powerful of all the protective antioxidant foods. The US Department of Agriculture has calculated the Oxygen Radical Absorbance Capacity, or ORAC, value – a measure of the protective value of foods – at 5,770 units per 100g, compared with 2,000 for raisins, blueberries and blackberries, and 980 for a plateful of Brussels sprouts. A handful of prunes provides the optimum protection of 5,000 ORACS a day.

RADISHES

Radishes are part of the *Cruciferae* family, like cabbage, broccoli and Brussels sprouts, and as such they contain glucosilinates and other sulphurous compounds that are valuable for those at risk from cancer. But it is for gall-bladder and liver problems that herbalists have found this delicious vegetable most useful. Radish juice has a powerful effect on the gall-bladder, making it contract and pump more bile into the stomach. It's this increase in bile that improves the digestion of fats, which is probably why radishes are so popular in France as a pre-dinner nibble. If you've never tried the traditional French snack of hot radishes dipped in butter, then salt, you've missed a wonderful treat.

Radishes are a rich source of other nutrients, too, as they contain potassium, calcium, sulphur, vitamin C, folic acid and selenium. But you can have too much of a good thing, and eating a whole bunch of radishes could irritate the liver, kidneys and gall bladder. For some people, the hot, peppery flavours can be a problem, and anyone with ulcers or gastric inflammation should treat them with caution. Like most of the *Cruciferae*, radishes can be affect the thyroid gland, and shouldn't be eaten by anyone with thyroid problems.

In the time of the pharaohs, radishes were regarded as a valuable food source – so much so that workers building the pyramids were paid in garlic, onions and radishes. In traditional Chinese medicine, they were listed in medical texts towards the middle of the seventh century. Although originally native to southern Asia, they're now widely cultivated throughout Europe, Britain, China and Japan. Surprisingly, they didn't reach the UK until the mid-1500s, when they were listed in an early herbal and recommended for their diuretic action and the prevention of gallstones.

Eat them as fresh as possible, while they're still young and crisp. And by the way, don't throw away the green tops; they're delicious and equally nutritious.

Raisins

The best-quality raisins and those with the most succulent flavour are produced from grapes which are allowed to dry naturally in the sun while still on the vine. In commercial production, they're laid out in bunches on the earth for about three weeks and turned regularly till they're dry. Australia and California are the major producers of raisins, and in both places they're dried in open-sided sheds to protect them against extremes of weather.

All the nutritional benefits of grapes are concentrated into raisins, making them a wonderful store of instant energy. Just 100g of raisins contain almost 70g of the natural sugars glucose and fructose. This makes them the perfect energy food for active people. Raisins are also ideal for anyone suffering from tiredness and exhaustion for any reason, whether it's anaemia, overwork, lack of sleep or chronic fatigue.

Unlike sweets and sugary drinks, they're rich in all sorts of other nutrients: fibre to help reduce cholesterol levels and improve bowel function; iron, with 100g providing more than twenty-five percent of the RDA for women; selenium; and a huge amount of potassium, which prevents fluid retention and helps reduce blood pressure. Raisins also contain small amounts of vitamin A and the B vitamins.

The combination of available energy and B vitamins means that raisins are helpful for anyone with depression, anxiety, stress and nervous tension.

Man has been drying fruits in the sun as a way of preservation for at least 5,000 years, and the Romans in particular included raisins in many of their medical prescriptions. When early settlers first travelled to the US, they took their dried fruits with them; today, raisins are firmly established as an American favourite. Many of the very finest raisins, especially the natural Thompson seedless, are now produced in California.

Organic raisins may not look so good, but aren't treated with sulphur or mineral oil. Both can be removed by washing in warm water.

Rosemary

In classical Greece, rosemary was revered as a remedy for depression and despondency, and its reputation was richly deserved. It is a true food for the mind and spirit – a perfect tonic for anyone who feels 'one degree under'.

Valued for its powers of 'remembrance', rosemary is both a tonic and stimulant of the brain's cortex. It eases general debility, improves memory loss, and reduces nervous tension. Modern research shows that it increases the amount of oxygen that individual cells are able to absorb, thus improving cell function and efficiency – which explains its effect on memory.

Originally a native of the Mediterranean, rosemary is a herb surrounded by myths and legends and highly favoured by mystics, magicians, old wives and sacred healers. One fable says that a rosemary bush will grow for thirty-three years and then die – as Christ did in his thirty-third year. Elizabethan couples carried rosemary on their wedding day as a sign of fidelity, and its fragrance was believed to ward off diseases like the plague.

Scientifically, the essential oils contained in rosemary are what provide many of its medicinal benefits. Borneol, linalool, esters and tannins are just some of the constituents which give it its antifungal and antibacterial properties. Rosemary tea makes a breath-freshening mouthwash, while the oil relieves joint pain and headaches as well as being a good insect repellant.

Used with lamb and chicken dishes throughout the Mediterranean, rosemary also contains camphor, limonene and rosemaricene; this is the reason it's anti-inflammatory. It also stimulates the gall bladder to increase the flow of bile to aiding fat digestion. In addition, the rosemaricene is a mild painkiller.

As a real treat, try hanging a bunch of rosemary sprigs under the hot tap of your bath to make the water truly invigorating and reviving to both body and spirit.

Sage

Sage is one of the cleansing, antiseptic and anti-inflammatory plant used by herbalists for menstrual problems, sweating and chest infections. Red sage, a Chinese relative, contains tanshinones, substances that stimulate the coronary circulation. It's also a powerful antiseptic, so try a teaspoon of chopped red sage in a glass of boiling water, cover it for ten minutes, and strain and cool before use.

Thujone is a phytoestrogen which helps to regulate periods and relieves many unpleasant menopausal symptoms, especially hot flushes. Because of its hormonal action, don't eat too much sage if you're breastfeeding, as it can reduce the flow of milk.

Its proper name is *salvia*, from the Latin *salvere*, which colloquially means 'to be in good health'. It's great with rich meats such as pork and venison, and is wonderful in the classic Italian dish of calves liver with sage. It's another herbal aid to fat digestion.

If stung or bitten by insects, rub the area with a few crushed sage leaves to relieve pain.

SARDINES

Fresh sardines cooked on a barbecue with a bowl of salad, a glass of wine and a chunk of real bread is a royal feast almost everyone enjoys on a Mediterranean holiday but hardly ever cooks at home. Fresh sardines are cheap to buy and widely available – even in supermarkets. They're rich in protein, iron and zinc, and are a very important source of vitamin D – without which you can't absorb calcium and build strong bones.

Like all oily fish, sardines supply the essential omega-3 fatty acids needed for proper development of the brain and all other nervous tissue.

Canned sardines are just as nutritious and have the added bonus of providing lots of calcium as, weight for weight, they're the only food which supplies more of this bone-building mineral than milk. That is, as long as you eat the bones. Mashed up with some Worcestershire sauce, balsamic vinegar and a squeeze of lemon juice and eaten with hot toast and a ripe tomato, they're a brain-, bone- and body-building feast.

Spinach

Spinach is exceptionally rich in folic acid, which is easily absorbed; 100g provides three-quarters of the adult daily requirement. This should put spinach firmly on the shopping list of every woman planning pregnancy or already expecting.

Cancer patients or those at risk from cancer, such as heavy smokers, should also eat lots of spinach. Cancer research has shown that spinach contains even more of the protective carotenoids than other dark-green or brightly coloured fruits and vegetables – even carrots (they may be rich in betacarotene, but not the other carotenoids). Two of these special chemicals, lutein and zeaxanthine, are major protectors of your eyesight, and spinach is one of the richest sources of both. The most common cause of impaired vision and blindness is age-related macular degeneration (AMD), and American studies have shown that people who regularly consume spinach and collard greens are much less likely to develop this debilitating illness than those who don't.

As every Popeye fan knows, spinach is rich in iron. But sadly, in this respect, generations of mothers who've tried forcing spinach down their children's throats have largely been wasting their time. The substantial amounts of iron and calcium in spinach are not easily available to the body, as spinach also contains oxalic acid. This combines with minerals that are excreted as insoluble salts. As spinach also contains uric acid, anyone with gout or arthritis should eat it sparingly.

This is an extremely versatile vegetable. The baby leaves can be eaten raw in salads; it makes an ideal snack just wilted for a few minutes and served with a little butter topped with a poached egg, or cooked without the addition of water, allowed to cool and served just warm, sprinkled with finely chopped raw onion, a squeeze of lemon juice, a dash of olive oil and a sprinkle of ground nutmeg.

Strawberries

There is a popular myth that anyone with arthritis should avoid strawberries because they are acidic; however, nothing could be further from the truth. In fact, strawberries are probably the nicest treatment you can imagine for this painful joint condition. These succulent fruits have an amazing ability to increase the body's elimination of uric acid: a substance that is highly irritating to inflamed joints.

Until the early 1600s, the only strawberries available in the UK and Europe were the tiny but succulent wild strawberry. Originally alpines, they were greatly valued as a delicacy and as a medicine. All the other strawberries that we enjoy today are descended from two American varieties.

Strawberries contain modest amounts of iron, but because of their extremely high vitamin C content, this is well-absorbed, which also makes them a good remedy for anaemia and exhaustion; 100g of strawberries provides almost twice your daily requirement of vitamin C.

Strawberries are an excellent source of pectin, a soluble fibre that helps eliminate cholesterol. Together with their high content of antioxidants, this makes strawberries a valuable weapon against heart and circulatory disease as well as a remedy for anyone already suffering from these diseases. There is also evidence of antiviral properties.

This is one medicine that doesn't need a spoonful of sugar to help it down. These wonderful berries should be eaten on their own, or at the start of a meal in order to achieve their therapeutic best. A daily bowl of strawberries is the cheapest and most delicious health insurance you'll ever buy.

Instead of sugar and cream, try adding a sprinkle of freshly ground black pepper. It may sound peculiar, but the heat of the pepper seems to draw out maximum flavour from the berries. If you want to be really adventurous, add a spoonful of balsamic vinegar as well – don't knock it till you've tried it.

Sweet potatoes

Sweet potatoes are a traditional lowland root crop in many tropical climates and were first brought to Europe by Columbus. He took them back to Spain, from whence they spread and enjoyed considerable popularity, but their appeal waned and they didn't become a common sight in Britain until the influx of immigrants from the Caribbean islands.

This created a new demand for the sweet potato, and many other delicious foods from the Caribbean, from the 1950s onwards. You'll find them today in every supermarket, street market and many corner shops. Sweet potatoes are often confused with yams, but in fact, they're a separate species; although many books describe them as alternative names for the same plant, the yam is nutritionally inferior.

Sweet potatoes are an excellent source of starch and, therefore, energy. They provide some protein, vitamin C, vitamin E and a huge amount of carotenoids, including betacarotene. It is these and the other phytochemicals in the tubers that make them such a powerful anti-cancer food. A mere 100g a day can dramatically reduce your risk of lung cancer – and this is even more important if you are a smoker or ex-smoker.

They're an extremely versatile vegetable and are wonderfully healthy for children and adults alike. A good way to introduce them to your family is to peel and cube a sweet potato and cook it together with ordinary potatoes, drain, mash with a little butter or olive oil and some grated nutmeg. They're equally delicious mashed together with parsnip or swede, and they're great just roasted in a medium oven, brushed with olive oil, and sprinkled with black pepper.

Surprisingly, they make an interesting addition to homemade juices, and combine well with other vegetables and many fruits. One of my favourite combos is apple, carrot, celery and sweet potato – which tastes better than it sounds.

Tea

Nutritionally, tea contains useful quantities of vitamins E and K and small amounts of the B vitamins. It's an important source of the trace elements manganese (essential for growth, bone-building and the function of hormones and enzymes) and fluorine (essential for strong bones and teeth and protective against tooth decay). In small quantities, the astringent tannins in tea are antibacterial and help with food poisoning and other stomach infections. The tannins are also good for eye problems; a used tea bag dipped in cold water and placed over closed eyes for ten minutes gives instant relief for sticky, itchy and tired eyes.

By far the most exciting benefits of tea come from the bioflavonoids: natural plant chemicals which act as antioxidants, neutralizing the damaging free radicals that cause heart and circulatory problems. Two to four cups a day are necessary for this extra protection, and though green tea is richer in protective substances, our British brew also contains significant amounts.

When it comes to cancer prevention, green tea is certainly top of the list. Its rich content of antioxidants is only part of the cancer-prevention story, as latest research has revealed another amazing chemical called EGCG, a substance known to slow the growth of tumours by stopping the development of new blood vessels which would otherwise supply them with the nutrients they need to develop. There are also interesting phenolic compounds that help strengthen blood-vessel walls – which makes tea a good drink if you've got thread veins, chilblains, varicose veins or cold hands and feet.

Trouble concentrating? Have a cup of tea. Psychologists have found that something in tea (and it's not the caffeine) improves concentration and speeds up the learning process. This benefit of tea is especially marked when you're trying to concentrate on more than one job at a time. So, if you're multi-tasking, maybe a cuppa is all you need to keep your mind on the job(s).

Tomatoes

The ancestral home of the tomato is the western coast region of South America, stretching from Ecuador to Peru and Chile. Even in the high mountains, wild varieties abound. and these are cherry tomatoes: the forerunners of all modern varieties.

The first domestication probably happened in Mexico, and tomatoes were introduced to Europe by the Spanish during the sixteenth century, after which they rapidly rampaged across southern Europe. As members of the *Solanaceae* family, which includes the deadly nightshade, they were treated with suspicion at first, but soon achieved their rightful place as a delicious and health-giving food.

Tomatoes are extremely rich in antioxidants, especially carotenoids such as betacarotene and lycopene, as well as vitamins C and E, making them good protectors of the cardiovascular system and against some forms of cancer. They're also extremely low in sodium and quite rich in potassium, so they are helpful in conditions such as high blood pressure and fluid retention.

There should always be a few cans of tomatoes in your cupboard, as they lose very little of their nutritional value during canning and are a great standby for instant high-nutrient sauces. A ripe tomato contains more than 200 volatile compounds that make up its unique taste and smell. Green tomatoes, however, contain a chemical called tomatine, which may trigger migraine attacks. It's also destroyed by cooking, but remains in quite high amounts in the pickled green tomatoes popular in the US.

A highly important recent discovery has been the role of lycopene, a carotenoid present in ripe tomatoes. This nutrient is known to protect men against prostate cancer – a much less common disease in Mediterranean countries where six to eight ripe tomatoes a day is the average consumption.

Interestingly, processed tomatoes contain far more lycopene than fresh ones, so tinned tomatoes, tomato sauce, ketchup and sun-dried tomatoes are extremely important, as they also protect men and women against heart disease.

Turmeric

Turmeric, a member of the ginger family, is native to India and China. It's grown for its root, which is used as medicine and as the most common flavour and colour in Chinese and other Far Eastern cooking. Popular for centuries, this essential ingredient of curry powder is key to successful Asian vegetarian food – particularly lentil recipes.

Indian Ayurvedic practitioners prescribe it for eyesight, rheumatism, arthritis and also liver problems. Today's scientists are fascinated by its powerful antioxidant and protective properties, which appear to work just like the non-steroidal anti-inflammatory drugs. In addition, this spice is now thought to have powerful cancer-preventive properties, with one huge advantage: there are no side effects.

Turmeric is one spice that should be a regular part of day-to-day eating, providing substantial amounts of the highly protective and immune-boosting antioxidants and the potentially cancer-preventive effects of curcumin, one of its natural constituents.

VENISON

Unfortunately, childhood memories of Bambi put lots of people off this delicious and healthy meat. But venison is making a comeback. Though it's more often farmed than wild, the flavours and texture are superb when the meat is properly dressed and hung.

Nutritionally, venison contains only a third of the calories and half the fat of beef, and even less of both than chicken, so it's genuinely a healthy option. It's also an excellent source of protein, iron and B vitamins, and even when it's farmed, it is much less likely to contain antibiotics, growth hormones and many other unwanted residues.

Prime cuts should be cooked very hot and medium-rare. Otherwise, marinate before cooking in red wine, oil and herbs (common in Europe and the UK), or buttermilk (an American favourite). When travelling in Wyoming, I also sampled one American hunter's campfire recipe cooked in coffee and cider vinegar, but nothing compares with traditional English venison hotpot, cooked slowly with lots of vegetables.

WALNUTS

Walnuts are one of the most ancient of all recorded foods. Archaeologists in southwest France have found fossilized walnut shells that were roasted more than 8,000 years ago. Engraved clay tablets dating from 2,000 BC showed walnuts growing in the hanging gardens of Babylon, and both the ancient Greeks and Romans treated them as a royal food and enshrined them in their mythology.

The most widely grown variety is the English walnut, which in fact originated in Persia and got its name from the English seafarers who carried them as cargo to trade around the world. The other variety is the black walnut, native to North America but seldom grown commercially. California produces the vast majority of the world's walnuts, but these are all English walnuts introduced commercially in 1867.

Walnuts are a wonderful health-giving and nutritious snack food, providing protein, slow-release energy, potassium, magnesium, copper, zinc, and vitamins B_6 and E. But the most important constituent is the oil. They have seven times more polyunsaturated than saturated fat, and the polyunsaturates are an important source of essential fatty acids which, combined with their antioxidant properties, make them ideal for anyone with heart or circulatory disease, raised cholesterol or high blood pressure. Scientific studies in the US and Spain have found that eating a handful of walnuts a day can significantly lower cholesterol levels.

If you're lucky enough to find wet walnuts – just after harvest and before the shells have dried out – they're a real delicacy. Although just as healthy when dried, eat them either straight from the shell or chopped into cakes, biscuits, salads and other recipes.

Walnut oil is fantastic for both flavour and health-giving properties and is produced in small quantities by local growers, especially in France and Italy. There are great variations in colour and flavour and it is expensive, but a drizzle into puréed parsnips, swedes and carrots, added to bread recipes or mixed with lemon juice as a salad dressing adds a truly delicious flavour.

WATERCRESS

Hippocrates described watercress and its medicinal values in 460 BC. He even built the world's first hospital next to a stream flowing with pure spring water so that he could grow fresh watercress for his patients. The Greeks and the Romans believed watercress was a cure for madness (though taking it mixed with vinegar didn't do much for Nero). The watercress you eat today is identical in every respect to that eaten by Hippocrates, Nero and even Henry VIII.

Thanks to its high vitamin C content, it has been used since the 1500s to prevent scurvy, but there's more to this nasturtium family member. Both watercress and nasturtiums contain a benzyl mustard oil that is powerfully antibiotic but, unlike conventional antibiotics, it's kind to your friendly gut bacteria. Eating watercress and nasturtium flowers strengthens your resistance and fights chest and urinary infections.

Dr Stephen Hecht, professor of cancer prevention at the University of Minnesota, has studied the importance of watercress as a preventer of lung cancer in smokers. The best way to avoid lung cancer is to stop smoking, but those who can't should make sure that they eat a large bunch of watercress every day. These peppery-tasting leaves contain a unique chemical, phenethyl isothiocyanate, which helps neutralize the important tobacco-specific lung carcinogen NNK. This extraordinary protective chemical, also known as gluconasturtiin, is only released from watercress when it is chewed or chopped.

Add all this to the fact that watercress is also a useful source of iodine – essential for the proper functioning of the thyroid gland – and you'll understand why it isn't just a garnish on top of the steak, but a nutritious, protective and important food which should be eaten in generous quantities by everybody.

Always wash watercress thoroughly in plenty of running water to remove any residual grit or bacteria. It makes great soup, wonderful sauce to go with fish, is delicious in salads and turns a mundane sandwich into a taste sensation.

WHEAT

Wheat is a vitally important staple food in the Western diet. The majority of wheat ends up as flour and, finally, bread. Although bread consumption is declining, it still accounts for a quarter of all the protein in the British diet. One hundred years ago, up to three-quarters of the population's protein came from bread.

In addition to protein, wheat provides energy, B vitamins and minerals, but it doesn't contain vitamins A, C or B_{12}. For the real taste of wheat, just compare a fresh loaf made from organically grown, wholegrain flour with nothing added but a pinch of salt and fresh yeast, with the white, cotton-wool, full-of-additives variety made from refined flour that has come from the agribusiness – this flour is from wheat grown on artificially fertilized and monocropped soil and sprayed with pesticides, insecticides and fungicides.

Although refined wheat flour is fortified with some lost nutrients, zinc, magnesium, B_6, pyridoxine, vitamin E and fibre are not replaced.

People with coeliac disease cannot eat wheat as it contains gluten, and there are others who don't tolerate this cereal very well. In fact, however, few of those claiming wheat allergy actually have it; it's more likely to be an intolerance often due to over-consumption, as in recent years pasta, pizza and burgers in buns have come to dominate our eating habits.

It's a shame that we can't eat more of the same foods our ancestors did. A centuries-old British dish called frumenty was the perfect meal for millions of farm labourers in years gone by: whole wheat grains were baked overnight in the ashes of the fire (which burst open the grains) and then set into a thick jelly, which was eaten with milk, spices, honey, currants or raisins.

The wheatgerm left behind when white flour is milled is a rich source of the vitamin B complex and vitamin E, which makes it an excellent food supplement, especially for invalids and convalescents.

WINE

When the French raise a glass of wine in a toast, they say *à votre santé* – 'to your health' – and those French certainly know a thing or two about the health benefits of booze. Red wine is one factor in the Mediterranean Diet that is known to protect against heart disease.

In most parts of the world as well as France, the drinker's toast is to their companion's good health – *saluté, skøl, prost, lekhayyim* – but here in the UK it's more likely to be an uninspiring 'cheers' or 'bottoms up'. That's a pity, because sensible amounts of wine are extremely beneficial and there's nothing new in that. Our most ancient ancestors discovered the art of fermentation and used their alcoholic drinks for the relief of pain. The ancient Greeks and Romans added herbs and spices to wine for medicinal purposes, and even the Bible is littered with references to the medical properties of alcohol.

French scientists have shown that men drinking moderate amounts of red wine on a regular basis have thirty percent less risk of death from all causes than heavy drinkers or total abstainers. Red grapes are an extremely rich source of natural antioxidants known as phenolic compounds, and these are known to be protective against a wide range of heart and circulatory diseases. These wines are often matured in oak casks, so they absorb even more of the natural antioxidants from the wood.

There's a good reason to enjoy Chardonnay, Sauvignon Blanc, Pinot Grigio and all the delicious white wines, too: they may be good for your lungs. Dr H Schunemann from the University of Buffalo, New York, has been studying lung function. Volunteers were questioned about their alcohol consumption, and after allowing for lifestyle, height, weight, eating habits and smoking, those drinking wine rather than other alcoholic beverages had healthier lungs. The white-wine-drinkers had the best lungs of all.

Yogurt

Yogurt in some form or other has been made since time immemorial. The ancient Bedouin found that the combination of heat and movement (and, obviously, a few good bacteria) fermented the milk in their goatskin bags. The resulting yogurt then kept for days.

Most commercial yogurts start out as pasteurized milk inoculated with cultures of beneficial bacteria such as *Lactobacillus acidophilus* or *bulgaricus*, *Bifidobacteria* or *Streptococcus thermophilus*. Yet many yogurt products are then pasteurized again and contain none of the live and beneficial organisms that give yogurt its unique properties.

Live, or 'bio' yogurts contain health-giving bacteria which synthesize B vitamins, biotin, folic acid and B_{12}. They increase absorption of calcium and magnesium, and keep your bowels regular. These 'good bugs' also attack and destroy the 'bad guys' that cause food poisoning.

Because antibiotics kill all bacteria, good and bad, they should always be taken with a daily carton of live yogurt to help prevent diarrhoea. Yogurt also actively encourages the synthesis of B vitamins, thus helping to prevent the depression that commonly follows antibiotic therapy.

Yogurt is an excellent source of calcium. One 150g carton provides 210mg – well over a quarter of the minimum daily adult requirement – and for weight-conscious women, low-fat varieties contain even more, at 285mg per 150g pot. Yogurt also supplies small traces of vitamin D, which is essential for the absorption of calcium, making it an even more important source.

Veterinary scientists have found that the 'probiotics' – good bugs – present in yogurt produce enzymes that are absorbed directly through the gut wall, which strengthens the immune defences.

A daily live yogurt is a huge health bonus. Choose a plain variety and add your own fruit to avoid sugar, preservatives and other chemicals.

2

vitamins & minerals

It's less than a century since these essential nutrients were discovered, yet today, shelves groan under a vast array of vitamin and mineral supplements. Do you really need them? For some people, the answer is yes – and there's nothing wrong with a daily multivitamin. However, the key to good health is to get everything you need from food, which is why this section includes a selection of the most important life- and health-enhancing nutrients.

Calcium

Calcium is vital for the formation and continuing strength of bones and teeth. This is of even greater importance during pregnancy, breastfeeding, childhood and for teenagers. In later life, women are at risk of osteoporosis (brittle-bone disease) caused by too little calcium in the diet and poor absorption.

Protecting bones begins in childhood, with a diet that contains calcium-rich foods. Encourage children to be active, play sport, get plenty of fresh air and sunshine; as you get older, these activities become even more important. Pregnant and nursing mothers need a good store of calcium. During your thirties, make a super effort to keep up some sort of regular exercise regime. It should be weight-bearing, to strengthen the bones, like tennis, dancing, keep-fit, walking or even energetic housework.

During menopause, women need extra calcium with vitamin D. Calcium also helps relieve the symptoms of PMS, helps prevent muscle cramp and is important as a regulator of the heart rate and blood-clotting.

A glass of milk, a carton of yogurt and 60g of cheese provide the 1,000mg of calcium you should get each day. Use low-fat versions and also eat plenty of tinned sardines (with bones), lots of greens and dried fruit, nuts, beans, and plenty of watercress and parsley. Your body needs sunlight to make vitamin

D, without which it can't absorb calcium, so get outdoors and remember to eat plenty of oily fish: the best nutritional source of vitamin D.

Dairy products contain the most easily absorbed calcium, though there's virtually none in butter, double cream or cream cheese. Some vegetables, like spinach and beet greens, contain oxalic acid which prevents the absorption of calcium, and wholegrain cereals, nuts and pulses contain phytic acid, which can also interfere with calcium absorption. Sprinkling bran all over your breakfast cereals seriously reduces the calcium absorbed from the milk for the same reason. Colas and other fizzy drinks contain phosphoric acid that seriously increases the amount of calcium eliminated by the body.

Although the RDA is 800mg per day, the optimum intake should be around 1,000mg, rising to 1,200mg during pregnancy and breastfeeding. The cheapest form of calcium supplements are made from calcium carbonate, but the body can't get much of the calcium from these products. It's far more effective to pay a little more for calcium citrate, from which your body extracts twice as much of the mineral.

Best sources
Cheese • Canned sardines • Tofu • Seaweed• Sesame seeds • Almonds • Figs • Yogurt • Semi-skimmed milk

FOLIC ACID

Folic acid, a member of the vitamin B group of nutrients, is found in a wide variety of foods and is best-known for its ability to prevent spina bifida in newborn babies. Unfortunately, it's the first three months of pregnancy that are crucial in the development of the baby's spine and when having adequate folic acid is so important. Many women don't realize that they are pregnant until the second or third month. In spite of the wide availability of folic acid, few people manage to get the 200 micrograms they need each day from their diet. Folic acid is also needed for the body's production of healthy red blood cells.

Latest research shows that it also plays a key role in the prevention of heart disease by controlling the amount of homocysteine in the blood. High levels of this naturally occurring chemical are known to be a factor which increases the risk of fatal heart attacks. Anaemia may be caused by getting too little folic acid and a supplement of 200 micrograms a day can soon help improve the condition and overcome the symptoms of severe tiredness.

After the menopause takes place the blood levels of homocysteine tend to increase, with a related increase in the risk of osteoporosis. For this reason it is extremely important for any women not having periods (for whatever reason) to make sure they eat a regular selection of folic-acid-rich foods. It's not advisable to take large amounts of folic acid – more than 500 micrograms daily – for long periods without discussing this with your GP, as at this level it may mask the symptoms of pernicious anaemia. Folic acid can also interfere with medicine taken for epilepsy, so epileptics must also talk to their doctor before taking it.

It's always best to take folic acid supplements together with food as this improves absorption. Alcohol, the pill, aspirin, anti-inflammatory drugs and medicines for non-insulin dependent diabetes can all interfere with the absorption of folic acid.

Best sources

Liver (but not to be eaten in pregnancy) • Fortified cereals • Beetroot • Brussels sprouts • Peanuts (fresh, unsalted) • Garbanso (black-eyed) beans • Spinach

Iron

Iron is one of the most important of all nutrients; without it, your body can't make haemoglobin, the substance that gives blood its red colour. It's haemoglobin that transports oxygen via the blood to every living cell in the body. As well as circulating in the blood, iron is also stored in the liver and other organs, and is available to make up for day-to-day variations in the amount of iron in the diet. Unfortunately, most women of child-bearing age and forty percent of schoolchildren do not get enough iron from their food and are consequently likely to become anaemic, one of the commonest nutritional disorders.

The iron RDA is 14mg, but this is set at around ten times the actual amount you need, because iron is poorly absorbed from most foods. Women need twice as much as men to compensate for their monthly blood loss, and they need even more during pregnancy to make sure that enough is passed to the baby and stored by the mother in preparation for breastfeeding.

Iron from animal sources is better absorbed than that from all other foodstuffs, and all iron is better absorbed in the presence of vitamin C. A glass of fresh orange juice with breakfast and plenty of fresh fruits, vegetables and salads spread throughout the day can make a substantial difference to the levels of iron in the blood.

A number of factors make it even more difficult for

your body to extract iron from food. Tannins from tea are an important factor, especially in older people whose diets may be poor and who tend to drink large amounts of strong tea. Wholegrain cereals, peas, beans and cocoa contain plenty of iron, but this is poorly absorbed because they also have high levels of phytates, which reduce absorption. Bran and high-bran cereals act in the same way. Although spinach is a very rich source of iron, you'd have to eat a kilo to get as much of the mineral as you would from 100g of beef.

Excessive fatigue, hair loss, pale skin and gums, feeling tired, headaches and shortness of breath are all signs of iron deficiency.

Natural supplements such as ferrous gluconate are less likely to cause digestive problems. One of my favourites is Spatone Iron (plus), a naturally occurring Welsh mineral water with a well-absorbed iron content. Conveniently packed in 20ml sachets, each one provide your daily need of absorbed iron at £6.49 for a month's supply. Do not exceed 15mg per day without professional advice. If you think you may be anaemic, see your GP to establish the underlying cause.

Best sources
Seaweed • Pheasant • Lambs liver • Beef • Sardines • Mussels • Brazil nuts • Balti vegetable curry

Potassium

Of all essential minerals, potassium is probably the least understood by the general public, but it is absolutely essential for many reasons. It is needed to maintain the balance between acids and alkalis in all body fluids and cells – a balance that is vital for survival. Potassium also plays a key role in the transmission of nerve impulses throughout the body, and in the prevention of calcium being lost in the urine. The other major function of this mineral is to promote muscle activity and prevent cramp, and it's in this area that most people will have heard about its importance.

Athletes have always been plagued by cramp. Until recently, the common perception was that cramp was caused by the amount of salt lost through sweating. Yet not only is salt ineffective in the relief or prevention of cramp, but it also increases the risk of high blood pressure, strokes and heart disease. Moreover, excessive salt intake causes oedema: the swelling of the hands, feet and legs due to fluid retention.

We're now used to seeing tennis players munching on bananas in the middle of a match, and footballers and other professional athletes packing them in their sports kits. This is because bananas supply easily digestible carbohydrates for energy and loads of potassium to prevent cramp and keep their muscles working efficiently.

Excessive consumption of sodium in any form, taking water tablets (diuretics), cortisone medication and too much alcohol can all reduce potassium levels. All fruits and vegetables, as well as instant coffee and red wine, contain potassium. But boiling your vegetables halves the content, as the mineral ends up in the cooking water, so make sure you use it in soups and gravies.

Blood loss, chronic diarrhoea or vomiting, diabetes, kidney disease or prolonged use of laxatives or diuretics can all cause potassium deficiency. This can be a particular worry in older people who tend to have a lower nutrient intake. Lack of potassium can cause muscle weakness, cramp, disorientation, mental confusion, depression and, if severe, heart attacks. Potassium supplements can help lower high blood pressure and reduce the risk of strokes, irregular heart rhythms and heart attacks.

The average adult needs 3,500mg of potassium daily. Supplements of 2,000mg to 3,000mg per day are adequate for the majority of people.

Best sources

Bananas • Dried apricots • Baked jacket potato • Prunes • Almonds • Dry-roasted peanuts • Stir-fry vegetables (courgette, Chinese cabbage, leeks, onion, garlic, spinach) • Tomato purée • Grilled chicken breast

Selenium

Selenium is a trace mineral, which means the body only needs tiny amounts each day – but a lack of it can be catastrophic. There's no official recommended daily amount, but most experts agree that 70 micrograms is the minimum we require. Worryingly, the average Brit today only gets around 30 micrograms, and this has serious implications.

Selenium is one of the major protective antioxidants that helps prevent damage to individual body cells. It's vital for the prevention of heart disease, and selenium deficiency is a major factor in the development of prostate cancer in men. Cancers of the lung and bowel are also thought to be associated with low intakes of selenium. Selenium is part of body's general defence mechanism, but it's also involved in the function of natural enzymes that regulate many of our bodily functions, including blood clotting and the protection of DNA – the genetic blueprint of every cell.

The amount of selenium that ends up in the food you eat depends firstly on how much there was in the soil in which the foods were grown or on which animals grazed, and secondly on the amount of processing to which the food has been subjected. Traditionally in the UK, most of our selenium was found in bread made from Canadian and North American wheat; the soil's selenium ended up in our bread. Now, thanks to the EU, our flour is made from European wheat with much lower selenium levels. What's more, our diets have become more and more reliant on processed and, therefore, deficient foods.

Virtually everyone in the UK needs to increase their intake of this vital mineral – particularly smokers; any man with prostate problems, poor fertility or a history of prostate cancer in the family; anyone with a family history of heart disease or any form of cancer; people with very poor diets; and vegans or vegetarians who don't pay attention to their nutrition. Selenium is also protective against many toxic chemicals as it combines with them and aids their removal from the body, so jobs that involve working with chemicals mean you need a higher intake.

Organically produced food has higher levels of selenium, and supplements are widely available in chemists and health-food stores. The mineral is best absorbed in the presence of vitamins A, C and E, but do not exceed a daily dose of 200 micrograms. It's present in most multivitamin and mineral pills.

Best sources

Brazil nuts • Wholemeal bread • Oily fish • Tuna, canned in oil • Sunflower seeds • Cooked mushrooms • Steak & kidney pie • Shrimp • Mixed nuts & raisins

Vitamin A

Vitamin A is essential for many different functions, including night vision and colour perception. It plays an important part in maintaining the body's natural defences by boosting immunity and resistance to viruses and bacteria. Another key function is the protection of mucous membranes – the linings of the mouth, nose, throat and lungs; without this vitamin, these tissues dry out and cannot perform their vital functions. Few people realize that vitamin A plays a key role in growth and bone development. It is required by men and women for fertility and reproduction. There is some evidence of its role in supporting the mechanisms of both taste and balance. Finally, vitamin A plays a key role in the growth and maintenance of healthy skin which keeps its elasticity; thus, as a bonus, it slows the development of wrinkles.

Because vitamin A is fat-soluble, the main sources are foods also containing some fats and oils. For this reason, it's essential to include fats, oils and the good food sources in the diet to make sure you get enough of this nutrient and that the body is able to absorb it. Anti-cholesterol drugs, antacid indigestion remedies and zinc deficiency can also reduce levels of vitamin A.

The body gets its supplies of vitamin A directly from foods containing it and indirectly through the conversion of betacarotene. Betacarotene is the brightly coloured yellow pigment found in foods such as carrots, apricots, sweet potatoes and most dark-green leafy vegetables, especially spinach.

The amount of vitamin A required each day is 800 micrograms. Although liver, oily fish, butter, cheese, carrots, vegetables and even milk offer substantial amounts, many people fail to get the minimum RDA, putting their health at risk. This is especially true of young women following extreme weight-loss diets.

The body stores surplus amounts of vitamin A in fatty tissues like the liver, so excessive doses can be extremely toxic. Never exceed the recommended dose of pills containing vitamin A and don't eat extremely rich sources such as liver more than a couple of times a week. Pregnant women should avoid vitamin A supplements and liver completely. Headaches, nausea, peeling itchy skin, hair loss and bone deformities can result from overdosing.

Cancer prevention is one of the major roles of vitamin A, but it's useful for people with chronic respiratory illness such as asthma and bronchitis.

Best sources
Liver • Carrots • Spinach • Butter • Eggs • Cheddar cheese • Dried apricots • Sweet potatoes

VITAMIN B$_6$ (PYRIDOXINE)

You need just 2mg of B$_6$ per day, but in spite of this nutrient being found in a large range of foods, it's quite common for people, especially women, to get less than the RDA in their diet. More importantly, larger intakes than the RDA can result in the reduction, prevention and even cure of a number of health problems. B$_6$ is essential for many chemical reactions that enable the body to use proteins and amino acids. It has a role in normal brain function, is important for red blood cells and the correct balance of the body's chemical make-up. B$_6$ is also a part of the body's system responsible for the excretion of water and the mechanism that produces energy from food. It protects against some types of anaemia and helps in stress control.

The best-known function of B$_6$ is the relief of PMS, thanks to its effect on hormone balance. It eases fluid retention, prevents mood swings, can dramatically improve depression and reduces episodes of aggressive behaviour in the days leading up to a period. Another condition that responds well to B$_6$ therapy is carpal tunnel syndrome. This type of RSI problem affects the nerves of the hand as they pass through the tissues of the wrist and can cause severe pain, burning, tingling and loss of sensation of the fingers.

Research has shown that many people who suffer chronic depression have low circulating levels of vitamin B_6 in their blood. My colleagues and I would certainly advise it for anyone with long-term depression. The whole of the central and peripheral nervous system needs adequate supplies of B vitamins; this group of nutrients is also helpful for the relief of chronic fatigue and Tired all the Time syndrome. In these instances, a B-complex tablet that includes B_6 is an invaluable part of holistic treatment.

Vitamin B_6 is excreted the same day you get it, so it's essential to have regular intakes. Anyone on high-protein diets, vegans, vegetarians, the elderly, women taking the pill or HRT, alcoholics and people with very low calorie intakes for any reason, need a B_6 supplement. This is also the case if you're taking penicillin, immunosuppressants or if you smoke.

Excessive amounts of B_6 can cause neurological problems including numbness of the hands and feet, clumsiness and general inflammation of the nerves; if this happens, stop taking the supplement immediately. These side effects have been reported at doses as low as 50mg a day, but in general, the safe upper limit is 250mg daily. I recommend starting at a dose of 50-100mg daily.

Best sources
Calves liver • Grilled herring • Turkey • Wheatgerm • Bananas • Wholemeal bread • Fresh unsalted peanuts

Vitamin B_{12}

B_{12} is part of the vitamin B complex which is essential for the prevention of pernicious anaemia. The RDA is only 1 microgram, which is easy to obtain from meat, fish, poultry, eggs, cheese and all animal-based foods. It is absent from virtually all plant foods except yeast extracts and fermented soy products, although it is often added to fortified breakfast cereals. For this reason, vegetarians and especially vegans should always take a daily supplement.

In order for the body to utilize B_{12}, a substance called the 'intrinsic factor', produced by the lining of the stomach, is essential, and the failure to produce enough is a common cause of pernicious anaemia. This condition used to be fatal, but it was first treated successfully with injections of liquidized raw liver – the richest source of B_{12}. In modern medicine, B_{12} itself can now be injected.

This vitamin is also needed for the production of a fatty substance called myelin, which forms a protective sheath covering all the nerves in the body. Deficiency of B_{12} reduces the amount of myelin, and as this is needed for the rapid transmission of nerve impulses, it can also result in serious neurological problems. Another function of this nutrient is the production of special enzymes which work together with folic acid. This means that vitamin B_{12} is also an essential requirement for the normal growth of babies during pregnancy and breastfeeding.

Enough vitamin B_{12} is stored in your liver to last around two years, but unless you continually replace what you're using, the reserve runs out, your bone marrow doesn't make enough healthy blood cells and the consequence is anaemia. Chronic fatigue, pale skin (especially inside the eyelids), loss of concentration, short-term memory, mood swings, sore tongue, loss of appetite, nausea, breathlessness and general weakness of arm and leg muscles can all be signs of B_{12} deficiency. Although the RDA is only 1 microgram, it's sensible to aim for 2 micrograms for children under 12, 3 micrograms for over-12s, and 5 micrograms for adults. As B_{12} is best absorbed in the presence of other vitamins, it's more effective as part of a multivitamin and mineral supplement than taken singly, unless prescribed by your health practitioner. The contraceptive pill, sleeping pills, some anti-diabetic drugs and excessive amounts of alcohol can all reduce absorption.

Best sources

Liver • Duck • Roast beef sandwich • Grilled plaice • Scrambled eggs • Vegetarian Cheddar • Soya cheese • Marmite

Vitamin C

Vitamin C is probably the best-known of all vitamins. Though it's by far the easiest to get in your diet, most people barely get enough each day. Vitamin C is a water-soluble vitamin found in virtually every variety of fruit and vegetable, although it is commonly linked with citrus fruits. It is a powerful antioxidant that protects every cell from damage caused by the free radicals that are by-products of pollution and natural chemical processes. A key benefit of this vitamin is the way in which it increases natural resistance to infection.

The RDA is 60mg, and while this is enough to prevent scurvy, none of the real nutrition experts believe it's anywhere near enough to promote the best-possible health. You'll get your daily allowance from a glass of orange juice, a kiwi fruit or 85g (3oz, of strawberries. For serious protection against flu, coughs and colds (an essential for smokers), avoiding cataract problems, fighting off cold sores, and to stimulate wound-healing after accidents or surgery, you need a minimum of 250mg daily – ideally 1,000mg or more.

Blackcurrants, papaya, green peppers and all green leafy vegetables are excellent sources, but for most people, a daily supplement could be the cheapest and best health insurance. Many studies have shown that vitamin C protects against infections.

The body cannot store large amounts of vitamin C, so you really need it on a daily basis. Professor Gladys Block, one of the world's leading experts on health and nutrition, says she aims for a minimum of 250mg each day, but for therapeutic purposes, for smokers, athletes, anyone in their 60s or routinely taking soluble aspirin to protect their heart, 500mg to 1,000mg is the optimum level. It's also important for women on the pill and anyone on long-term antibiotics or steroid drugs to increase their vitamin C intake, both from food and supplements.

Vitamin C is best absorbed when eaten with good sources of bioflavonoids. Bioflavaonoids are a large group of naturally occurring chemicals found in many fruits and vegetables. In citrus fruits, for example, they are present in the pith between the skin and the flesh. The highest concentrations are in the most brightly coloured produce. Bioflavonoids improve the body's absorption of vitamin C, and this is helped even more if you eat foods containing calcium and magnesium.

Best sources

Strawberries • Papaya• Kiwi fruit • Green peppers (raw) • Oranges • Broccoli (cooked) • Blackcurrants (cooked) • Coleslaw (homemade)

Vitamin D

Vitamin D is the vital key to strong, healthy bones. Together with sufficient calcium, it's essential for your bones as, without it, the body cannot absorb calcium from food. In childhood, a lack of vitamin D prevents bones from hardening and causes rickets, a condition that leads to bone deformity, bow legs and disability. A lack of vitamin D in adults results in osteomalacia – softening of the bones. It doesn't matter how much calcium you get from your diet or supplements; without vitamin D, the end result will almost certainly be osteoporosis, causing loss of height and a greatly increased risk of fractures of the hip, spine and almost any other bone in your body.

The body can manufacture its own vitamin D and this takes place when skin is exposed to ultraviolet light from the sun. Vitamin D formed in this way is stored in the skin and slowly released into the blood, then converted into a hormone-like chemical in the liver and kidneys. It's this active form of vitamin D that the body needs to extract calcium from food. If you don't get enough sunshine on your skin – ten to fifteen minutes a day on arms, legs, and face without sun block; early morning or late afternoon is perfectly safe – and you're not eating sufficient of the vitamin D-rich foods, then you can't maintain strong bones or teeth.

Those at special risk are the elderly, vegetarians, vegans, breastfeeding and pregnant women, and anyone who spends little time outdoors during the summer. The Asian community is often at risk due to traditional clothing, diet and lifestyle. Anybody in these groups or with a family history or diagnosis of osteoporosis must take a vitamin D supplement. But be careful: vitamin D at ten times the daily need can be toxic to children; 25 times is dangerous for adults. Don't give more than a teaspoon of cod liver oil to the kids each day or exceed this amount during pregnancy. The official RDA is 5 micrograms but 10 micrograms daily is a much more sensible target to aim for, especially if you're over 60 and your diet is not a good source of vitamin D.

Few foods contain vitamin D, but this fat-soluble nutrient is abundant in oily fish. There are modest amounts in eggs and it is added to margarines. There is no vitamin D in any fruit, vegetables and other plant foods. Ten micrograms will be obtained from 1 teaspoon of cod liver oil, 45g of herring or kipper, 55g mackerel, 80g canned salmon or tuna or 135g canned sardines.

Best sources

Cod liver oil • Herring & kippers • Smoked mackerel • Sardines: grilled & canned • Grilled trout • Grilled salmon steak • Eggs

Vitamin E

Even though this fat-soluble vitamin is found in a wide selection of foods, many people do not get the RDA of 10mg from their normal diets. Generally, the body builds up its own stores of fat-soluble vitamins, but vitamin E is an exception – which is why it's so important to get adequate amounts on a regular basis.

Vitamin E is one of the most powerful of natural antioxidants and is essential for protecting the body from the damage done by free radicals. It's especially important for cell walls, skin, muscles, nerves, blood vessels and the heart. This vitamin is also believed to be important for fertility, and high doses have been shown to increase the number of sperm in men with low sperm counts. High doses of vitamin E (more than 200mg) should not be taken by anyone with high blood pressure or heart disease without advice from their GP.

Taking the pill, environmental pollution and the action of the unhealthy trans-fats in many margarines can all interfere with vitamin E levels. Cholesterol-lowering drugs and excessive intake of iron or copper can also lower the body's levels of vitamin E. For this reason, vitamin E supplements should be taken at least four hours apart from mineral supplements that include iron and copper.

The body's absorption of vitamin E is increased by vitamin C and the mineral selenium. Interestingly, many of the nuts and seeds rich in vitamin E are also good sources of selenium. Eating vitamin C-rich foods at the same time as those containing vitamin E helps ensure maximum absorption.

Vitamin E is protective against heart disease, some forms of cancer (especially of the lung) and, together with vitamin C, may be useful in the treatment of cataracts. Some long-term vitamin E studies have shown that the heart-protective benefits are better when high intakes of vitamin E come from food rather than just relying on supplements. This is probably because foods rich in vitamin E also tend to be those with high levels of other naturally protective antioxidants.

Loss of libido, low levels of stamina, varicose veins, piles, thread veins, repeated infections and slow wound-healing may all indicate a shortage of this essential vitamin.

Best sources

Wheatgerm oil • Avocado • Baked sweet potato • Wheatgerm • Sunflower seeds • Rapeseed oil • Hazelnuts • Blackberries • Tomato purée

ZINC

Zinc is a greatly ignored trace element that is essential for children's growth, wound-healing, healthy sex organs, reproduction, insulin production and natural resistance to disease. Zinc is also essential for the senses of taste and smell and it plays a role in the creation of a good appetite. Without adequate zinc, men are not able to produce sufficient sperm and may become infertile.

One of the best-known folklore aphrodisiacs is the oyster, and although most people scoff at the thought of any foods being actual aphrodisiacs, oysters are the richest of all sources of zinc. Casanova reputedly ate up to seventy a day, usually enjoying them in the bath with his latest conquest.

Brittle nails, especially with white flecks, are nearly always attributed to a lack of calcium. In fact, there's very little calcium in nails and the most common cause is a lack of zinc. Meat, shellfish, fish, cheese and eggs are all good sources, but although wholemeal bread, nuts, wholegrains and some vegetables contain reasonable amounts of zinc, it is difficult for the body to extract much of it, due to their content of other chemicals such as phytates and oxalic acid.

Taking the pill and long-term use of the antibiotic tetracycline, often prescribed for acne, also reduce absorption of this mineral. Vegetarians and vegans may be seriously short of zinc, and this is a worry as there are no readily available stores in the body which can make up for fluctuations in your daily consumption. This can be an important factor for children and nursing mothers, as they both need extra supplies – children for growth and repair of damaged cells and mums for the high content in their milk.

Acne, PMS, post-natal depression, loss of appetite, slow wound-healing, poor hair and nails, anorexia nervosa, slow growth in children, hyperactivity and loss of the sense of smell are all signs that extra zinc may be needed. Prostate health in men is highly dependent on adequate supplies of zinc, and a deficiency can lead to enlargement of the prostate and, especially when combined with selenium deficiency, a greater risk of prostate cancer.

The RDA is 15mg per day.

Best sources
Oysters • Calves liver • Sardines • Roast beef • Pumpkin seeds • Crab • Eggs • Cheese

Healing foods

Acne   Cabbage and its many relatives are all rich in sulphur.
Fennel stimulates the liver and improves fat digestion.
Garlic is a powerful antibacterial.

Anaemia   Chicory is a good source of iron.
Watercress contains iron, betacarotene and is highly cancer-preventive.
Dates provide iron for vegetarians.
Red meat provides the most easily absorbed form of iron.

Anxiety   Basil, camomile, lavender and rosemary contain soothing natural chemicals.

Arthritis   Avoid red meat. For rheumatoid arthritis: reduce dairy products and avoid potatoes, tomatoes, peppers, and aubergines as well as cucumbers.
Eat lots of oily fish, ginger and chilli.

Asthma   Onions, leeks and garlic contain powerful natural chemicals which improve breathing and relieve congestion.
Avocado is a rich source of vitamin E.
Watercress protects the lungs.

Bloating	Celery, parsley are cleansing and diuretic. Mint eases flatulence, improves digestion.
Blood-sugar Problems	Carrots, parsnip, swede, oats and beans all supply good slow-release energy from complex carbohydrates. Dried fruits produce instant energy and slower-release energy from apricot fibre.
Catarrh	Onions, leeks and garlic contain powerful natural chemicals which improve breathing and relieve congestion. Watercress protects the lungs. Oregano helps clear the sinuses.
Cholesterol	Garlic, chives and oregano all help to eliminate cholesterol. Oats, apples and pears are rich in cholesterol-lowering fibre. Dried beans are good sources of protein, fibre and energy.
Chronic Fatigue Syndrome	Basil, bay, lemon balm and sage improve mood and generate mental energy. Complex carbohydrates, cereals, pulses and root vegetables provide physical energy. Meat, poultry, fish, eggs and other dairy products provide essential protein.

Circulation Problems	Basil, chives, coriander and sorrel help stimulate circulation. Ginger and chilli have similar actions. Oily fish contains omega-3 fatty acids, while nuts and seeds provide vitamin E for a healthy heart and circulation.
Colds	Garlic, chives and leeks are antibacterial and help clear mucus. Rosemary, sage and thyme are all powerful antibacterials. Cinnamon and cloves help ease coughs. Pumpkin seeds and shellfish contain zinc to boost the immune system.
Cystitis	Garlic is antibacterial and antifungal. Dandelion leaf tea, celery and parsley are effective diuretics. Cranberry juice keeps the bladder healthy.
Depression	Basil helps ease the anxiety that so often accompanies depression; add it to salads and sandwiches. Hops are calmative and improve sleep quality; use as tea. Oats are rich in B vitamins. Bananas, liver and chocolate increase levels of tryptophan, a gentle mood enhancer.

Eczema   Pumpkins, red and yellow peppers, broccoli, and sweet potatoes provide masses of skin-essential betacarotene.
Wholegrain cereals contain B vitamins that help reduce stress.
Oily fish supply anti-inflammatory essential fatty acids.

Fever   An onion is ideal and effective. Baked one in its skin for 40 minutes then finely chopped and mixed in equal parts with honey; take a teaspoon every two hours.
Teas made from thyme, sage, oregano, marjoram are antibacterial and antiviral.
Garlic crushed with ginger and lemon juice is an excellent general fever remedy.
Lemon juice and hot water sweetened with honey makes a great fever medicine for children; give two or three cups during the day, and one at bedtime.

Fluid Retention   Parsley is a natural diuretic. Add generously to cooking, as a garnish and in salads. It is also excellent as a tea.
Celery is also gently diuretic. Use in juices as well as raw or cooked.

Frigidity   Assuming there are no underlying serious medical problems, many foods may help: avocados, nuts and seeds for vitamin E, fish and shellfish for iodine, eggs for iron and B vitamins, tropical fruit for sexually enhancing enzymes; also coriander, ginger and cayenne.

Gastritis   Sage is astringent and cleansing; drink two cups of sage tea daily.
Mint is an effective antacid and helps settle the stomach; use generously in cooking and drink as a tea after meals.
Cereals such as rice, couscous and oats soothe the digestive tract.
Live yogurt contains beneficial probiotic bacteria to improve digestion.

Hair Problems   Often the result of anaemia or thyroid problems. Can be helped by improving scalp circulation.
Eat grated horseradish in a sandwich.
Liver and red meat supply enormous amounts of iron and B vitamins to help with stress.
Fish and shellfish are good sources of iodine for the thyroid as well as many trace minerals.

Halitosis	Fresh, raw foods like apples, pears, celery and carrots help to protect against gum disease. All citrus fruits supply vitamin C for gum protection. Herbs like fennel, dill, mint and star anise are breath fresheners. Live yogurt maintains good digestion.
Headache	Rosemary, mint and basil are traditional remedies for the relief of stress and its accompanying headaches. Liver provides iron and B vitamins, both of which help to reduce stress. Eating regularly will help keep blood sugar on an even keel and prevent headaches caused by hypoglycaemia.
Heart Disease	Garlic lowers blood pressure and cholesterol as well as reducing the stickiness of the blood; eat at least one whole clove daily in food. Ginger, chilli and curry spices contain phytochemicals to improve circulation. Wholegrain cereals and all dried beans protect the heart by lowering cholesterol. Oily fish is heart-protective.

High Blood Pressure	Garlic lowers blood pressure and cholesterol as well as reducing blood stickiness. Eat at least one whole clove daily in food. A cup of parsley tea two or three times daily is a good diuretic which eliminates excessive fluid, lowering blood pressure.
Impotence	Zinc and selenium are vital. Oysters, pumpkin seeds and Brazil nuts are some of the richest sources. Ginger, chilli, Tabasco sauce, cloves, turmeric and all curry mixtures help improve the peripheral circulation.
Indigestion	A glass of mint tea sweetened with a little honey after each meal and at bedtime will help relieve heartburn. Fennel and anise seeds are excellent remedies; use to make a tea; drink a cup after each meal. Carrots are a traditional remedy for all digestive problems; best eaten puréed.
Infertility	Men should see the advice under impotence, but both men and women need an abundance of vitamin E. Eggs, oily fish and shellfish are all good sources of other nutrients important for female fertility; volatile oils in coriander are also important.

Influenza	Lemon balm helps to relieve headaches associated with flu and is antiviral. A mixture of hot mint and ginger tea with honey is a general soother. Turmeric and chilli stimulate circulation and boost recovery. Live yogurt's beneficial probiotic bacteria are mood-boosters. Wholegrain cereals and oats provide B vitamins which help avoid the normal depression following flu. Chicken soup contains soothing compounds.
Insomnia	Lettuce helps induce sleep. Milk, starchy foods, turkey and oily fish provide soporific tryptophans. Nutmeg is mildly hallucinogenic. Lime-blossom tea has a natural relaxant.
Joint Pain	Ginger and chillis relieve pain. Oily fish is anti-inflammatory.
ME	Basil, bay leaf, lemon balm and sage improve mood and generate mental energy, the first step on towards recovery. The next essential is physical energy from complex carbohydrates, cereals, pulses and root vegetables. Protein from meat, poultry, fish, eggs, dairy products is the final ingredient.

Memory Loss	Rosemary is an ancient herbal remedy. Dried fruits and complex carbohydrates provide slow-release sugar. Oily fish and pumpkin seeds supply essential fatty acids: vital for brain function. Garlic reduces cholesterol and improves blood flow to the brain. Sage enhances mental performance. Dried fruits provide quick and slow-release energy.
Menstrual	Liver supplies a rich iron content. Celery and parsley are both gentle diuretics and overcome fluid retention. Oily fish supply the anti-inflammatory effect of fatty acids. Dates provide extra iron. Bananas supply cramp-relieving potassium and PMS-fighting vitamin B_6.
Mouth Ulcers	Basil and rosemary supply calming essential oils. Starchy foods like pasta, rice, bread and potatoes provide brain-soothing tryptophan.

Nail Problems	Oysters and pumpkin seeds provide zinc. Olive oil can be rubbed in as a moisturizer.
Neuritis	Wholegrain cereals and red meat supply B vitamins. Oily fish provide protective essential fatty acids.
Night Sweats (Menopause)	All soy products and beans provide natural plant oestrogens. Bananas contain vitamin B_6.
Osteoporosis	Soy/soy products provide plant oestrogens. Dairy products, beans and peas supply calcium. Oily fish offer vitamin D.
PMS	Liver provides a rich source of iron. Celery and parsley are both gentle diuretics and help overcome fluid retention. Oily fish give anti-inflammatory fatty acids. Dates offer extra iron. Bananas supply cramp-relieving potassium and PMS-friendly vitamin B_6.
Prostate Problems	Oysters and pumpkin seeds supply vital zinc. Brazil nuts provide selenium.

Raynaud's Disease	Ginger, chillis, onions, leeks and garlic to stimulate blood flow and reduce its stickiness.
Restless Legs	A common cause of insomnia and fatigue, sometimes the result of iron deficiency. Chicory suppliese iron; the bitter flavour is also an excellent appetite stimulant. Watercress contains iron, betacarotene and is highly cancer-preventive. Dates are a good iron source for vegetarians. Red meat provides the most easily absorbed form of iron.
Seasonal Affective Disorder (SAD)	Basil helps the anxiety that often accompanies depression; add to salads and sandwiches. Oats are rich in B vitamins. Bananas, liver and chocolate are helpful in increasing levels of tryptophan, a gentle mood enhancer. These remedies only help to relieve the symptoms of SAD; exposure to daylight or a light box together with the herbal remedy Hypericum (St John's Wort) should be used for the best possible results.
Shingles	All citrus fruits and buckwheat provide bioflavonoids and vitamin C. Leeks and ginger help relieve pain.

Skin-ageing   Protect your skin with antioxidants by maintaining a regular consumption of prunes, blueberries, garlic, kale, cranberries, strawberries, spinach, avocado and broccoli. Dehydration causes skin damage, so drink 1.5 litres of water daily.

Stress   Basil, camomile, and rosemary all contain soothing natural chemicals.
Meat and poultry provide iron and a plentiful supply of B vitamins which help combat the debilitating effects of stress.

Tired all the Time Syndrome (TATT)   Basil, bay, lemon balm and sage improve mood and generate mental energy, the first step on the road to recovery. The next essential is physical energy that is derived from complex carbohydrates, cereals, pulses and root vegetables. Protein from fish, meat, and dairy products is the final ingredient.

Thyroid Problems   Underactive thyroid may be caused by lack of iodine. Seafish and shellfish are both good sources.

Tonsillitis   Pineapple and pineapple juice supply the healing enzyme bromelain.

Urinary Problems	Parsley, celery and dandelion leaves all contain natural diuretic chemicals. Cranberry juice and berries supply antibacterial protection against infections. Camomile tea contains soothing volatile oils.
Varicose Veins	Porridge, muesli, apples, pears and beans provide soluble fibre to prevent constipation. Wholemeal bread, brown rice and wholegrain cereals give insoluble fibre for bulk. Buckwheat provides protective rutin. Citrus fruits, blackcurrants, blueberries supply vitamin C and bioflavonoids. Liver, shellfish, pumpkin seeds, sardines and eggs supply zinc, another vein-protector. Safflower and olive oil, avocados, nuts and seeds provide vitamin E.
Viral Infections	Oily fish offer essential fatty acids. Spinach, sweet potatoes and carrots supply betacarotene for vitamin A. Chickpeas, wholegrain cereals and lean meat give protein, B vitamins and folic acid. All citrus fruits, cherries, berries and fresh vegetables provide vitamin C. Tomatoes offer immune-boosting lycopene. Nuts, seeds, olive oil, avocados give vitamin E. Shellfish and pumpkin seeds provide zinc. Bay leaves, marjoram, thyme, lemon balm contain antiviral volatile oils.

Index

Numbers in **bold** are main references.